WOUND CARE MANAGEMENT

for the Equine Practitioner

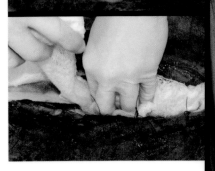

Dean A.
Hendrickson
DVM, MS

Made Easy Series
Teton NewMedia

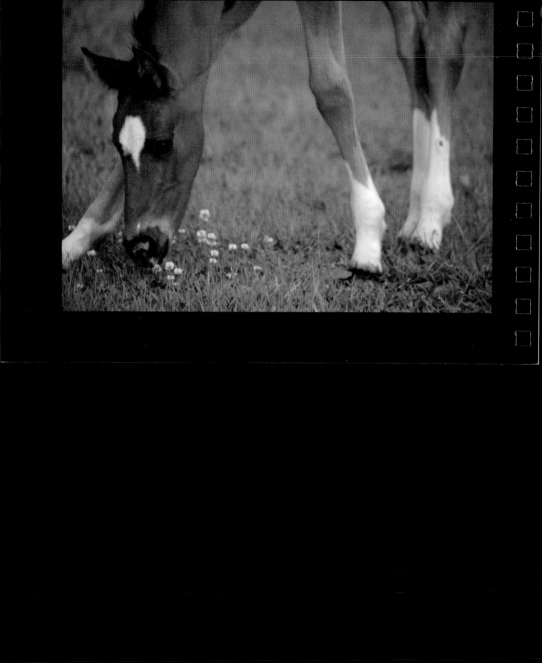

Wound Care

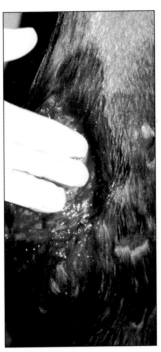

for the
Equine Practitioner

Dean A. Hendrickson, DVM, MS
Diplomate American College of
Veterinary Surgeons

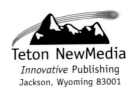

Teton NewMedia
Innovative Publishing
Jackson, Wyoming 83001

Executive Editor: Carroll C. Cann
Development Editor: Susan L. Hunsberger
Production & Layout: 5640 Design, www.fiftysixforty.com

Teton NewMedia
P.O. Box 4833
4125 South Hwy 89
Jackson, WY 83001
1-888-770-3165
www.tetonnm.com
www.veterinarywire.com

PRINTED BY ADVANCED LITHO PRINTING, GREAT FALLS, MT.

ISBN # 1-59161-021-4

Print number 5 4 3 2 1

   Library of Congress Cataloging-in-Publication Data

Hendrickson, Dean A.

   Wound care for the equine practitioner / Dean A. Hendrickson.

     p. cm. – – (Made easy series)

   Includes bibliographical references (p.).

   ISBN 1-59161-021-4 (alk. paper)

     1. Horses – – Wounds and injuries – –Treatment. I. Title. II. Made easy series
   (Jackson, Wyo.)

SF951.H495 2004

636.1'08971 – – dc22

                                          2004041271

Dedication

This book is dedicated first and foremost to my wife and children who put up with me working on the book when I should have been playing ball, going swimming, or just hanging around. You are my favorite people in the world, and you have made me a better person with your love and care for me.

It is also dedicated to all of the students and horse owners that have challenged me to be a better veterinarian. I hope that you will enjoy the book as much as I have enjoyed learning about wound care.

Dean A. Hendrickson

September, 2003

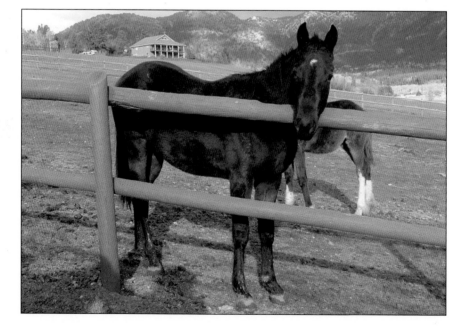

Acknowledgements

This book would not have been possible without a few key people. Thanks to Meredith Anderson for the prodding and encouragement to try some new techniques. Thanks to Judy Papen for the education on figuring out how to use some of the advanced wound care products. And finally the encouragement of Dr. George Rodeheaver in helping me to know that I could actually get this information down in print.

Drs. Luis Silva, Gayle Trotter, and Troy Trumble have supplied various figures. Thank you for helping out where I needed the help.

The CD layout was the idea of Lauren Javernick; thanks for all of your hard work.

And a special thanks to the people at Teton NewMedia, especially Carroll Cann, for all of your hard work and guidance.

Table of Contents

Wound Debridement 41

Section 3   Wound Exploration

Section 4 Primary Wound Closure

Section 5 Delayed Primary Wound Closure

Section 6 Second Intention Wound Healing

Section 8 Specific Wound Considerations

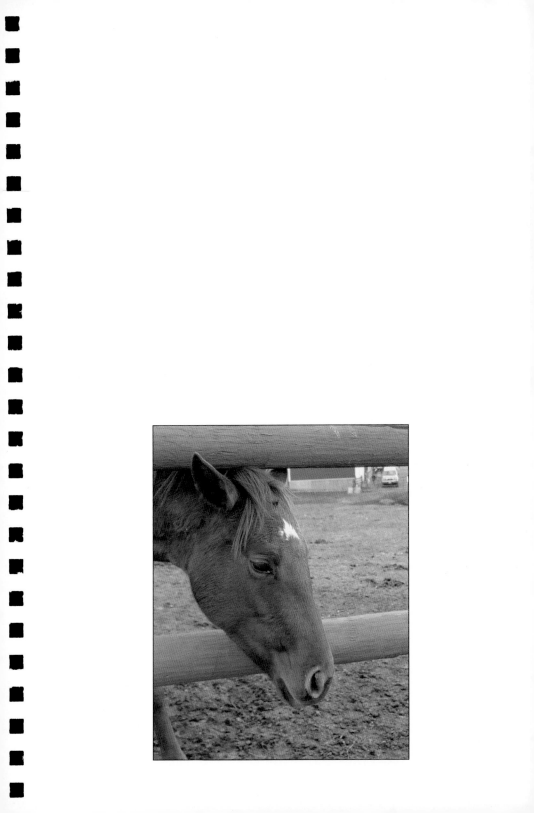

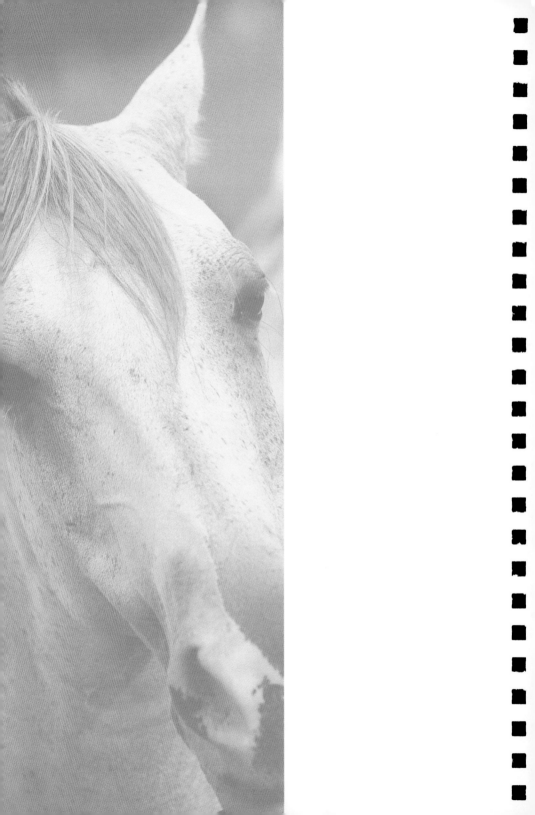

Section 1

Wound Care Dressings

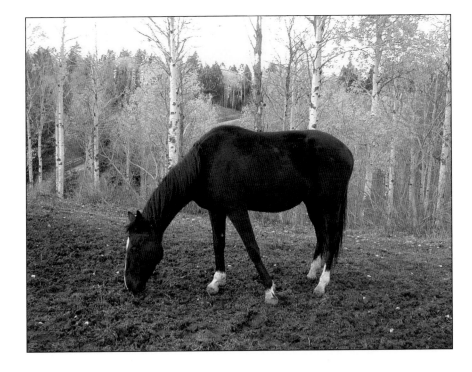

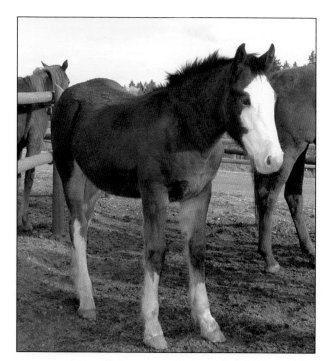

Introduction

Wound care is part of everyday practice for the equine practitioner. It can be either very frustrating or rewarding, and sometimes both, to try and provide the best functional and cosmetic outcome for our clients and patients. The goal of this book is to help veterinarians work with one of the most common ailments of the horse-wounds. This book will cover basic and some advanced wound care principles as general topics, along with specific wound considerations. There are many tried and true principles that will be discussed as well as some new and exciting principles.

Some Helpful Hints

Scattered throughout the text, you will find the following symbols to help you focus on what is routine and what may be really important:

✓ This is a routine feature or basic point for understanding the subject discussed.

♥ This is an important feature. You should remember this.

⚷ The key symbol will be used selectively to indicate a very important point to assist your understanding of the topic area.

✋ Stop. This does not look important, but it can really make a difference when trying to sort out unusual or difficult situations. It can be my opinion based on personal experience.

💣 Something serious will happen if you do not remember this, possibly resulting in injury or loss to the patient, and upset to the client.

⊙ A companion CD is available for purchase by calling 877-306-9793. The CD contains the full text, figures, and tables of this book formatted for easy search and retrieval. The CD symbol indicates that additional images of a topic are available on the CD.

This section will help the practitioner to identify the different types of wound dressings that are available.

✔ Wound care dressings include any therapy that can be used to treat a wound.

♥ Often these dressings are used in multiple layers providing distinct benefits for the desired outcome. Dressings can include anything from a simple non-adherent pad to a complex synthetic semi-occlusive pad and everything in-between.

♥ For many veterinarians, the number of dressings available can be overwhelming. It is important to recognize that most dressings have been designed for specific purposes.

⚷ In many cases, equine practitioners have traditionally used dressings for tasks they weren't designed for, in order to minimize the number of different materials needed. While this technique may work, it is likely that appropriate use of specific materials will provide a more satisfactory outcome. While the list could be very long, there are eight general dressing categories that will be discussed. In some instances, the same dressing could be included in more than one category.

Dressings Used for Cleaning and Prepping

✔ Many dressings have been used for cleaning and prepping. The purpose is often twofold: one to reduce the amount of debris, and the other to minimize risk of infection.

✋ The most commonly used dressings for cleaning and prepping are gauze dressings; however, not all gauze dressings are created equal (Figure 1-1). Gauze is available in both woven and non-woven forms. Each of the forms has positive and negative characteristics (Table 1-1). In general, woven gauze is better for cleaning and prepping than is non-woven gauze because of the loose weave and the inherent strength they provide.

💣 The superior prepping and debriding characteristics, while beneficial in some cases, are detrimental in others. One example is a wound that is clean and free of bacterial infection. When woven gauze is used to clean the wound, the superficial fibroblasts and epithelial cells are removed, retarding the healing process. In some cases, enough mechanical trauma ensues to increase the likelihood of infection. In summary, woven gauze is

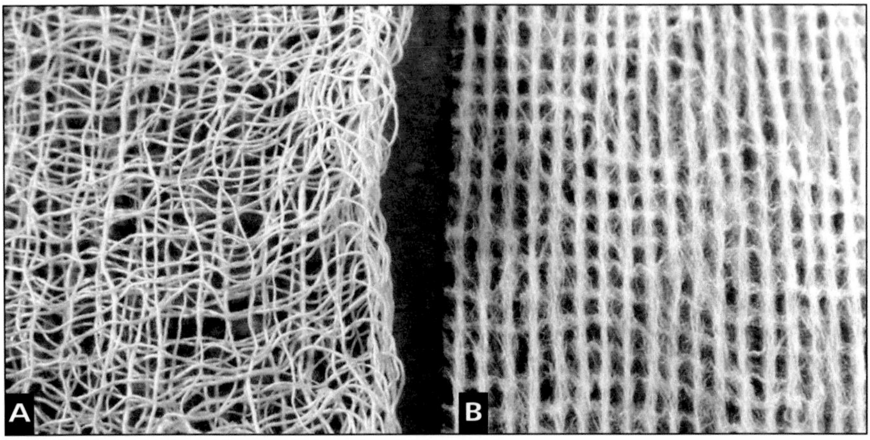

Figure 1-1 A. Woven and **B.** non-woven gauze.

Table 1-1 Woven -vs- Non-woven Gauze

WOVEN GAUZE	NON-WOVEN GAUZE
Made of 100% Cotton	Primarily Synthetic Blends
Moderate Lint Levels	Low Lint Levels
High Strength	Low Strength
Moderately Absorbent	Highly Absorbent
Vertical Wicking Ability	Horizontal Wicking Ability
Conformable	Resilient
Relatively Adherent	Less adherent
Moderate to High Loft or Bulk	Little Loft or Bulk
Superior Debridement Characteristics	Poor Debridement Characteristics
Superior Prepping Characteristics	Poor Prepping Characteristics

best used on normal skin when aggressive cleaning properties are needed. Non-woven gauze is best used for cleaning wounds and surgical sites where less mechanical trauma will occur with use.

✓ Cotton and foam applicators impregnated with some type of antiseptic are often used in human medicine to clean and prep an area. They are rarely used in horses due to the expense and the surface area involved in the preparation.

Dressings Used for Debridement

♥ Debridement can be achieved through various methods including sharp debridement, physical debridement, chemical debridement, autolytic debridement, and enzymatic debridement. Dressings are generally used to achieve physical and autolytic debridement. The methods of debridement will be more completely discussed in Section 2.

✓ Physical debridement employs the concept of removing contamination and devitalized tissue with a dressing using physical force (Figure 1-2). In most cases, woven gauze is used to perform this task (see Table 1-1). Woven gauze is more aggressive than non-woven gauze in removing both contamination and tissue. Large amounts of contamination or devitalized tissue will impede healing.

🖐 It is important to remember that in some cases, physical debridement is more traumatic than beneficial to the wound bed. Consequently the use of physical debridement should be carefully considered and used only when removal of tissue and contamination by physical force will ultimately lead to the best possible outcome.

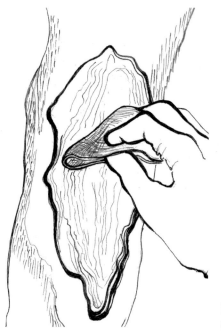

Figure 1-2 Drawing showing gauze debridement.

⌐ In most cases, sharp debridement should be used to begin the debridement phase, and less aggressive physical debridement used to finish the process.

♥ Autolytic debridement occurs when an appropriate dressing is chosen to maintain the proper moisture balance at the wound surface (Figure 1-3). The wound exudate is then left in contact with the wound, allowing better access of white blood cells and autologous enzymes to remove the devitalized tissue. Autolytic debridement requires a moist wound, and will only remove devitalized or diseased tissue, whereas physical debridement is nonselective. Calcium alginate and semi-occlusive foam dressings are examples of dressing types that are used for autolytic debridement.

✋ Autolytic debridement is more completely described in Section 2. Specific dressing types will be described in more detail in Section 6.

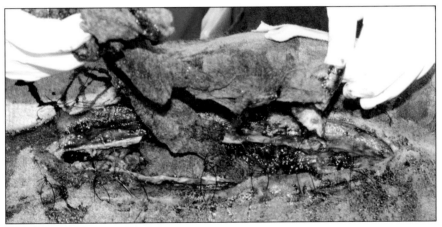

Figure 1-3 Wound over dorsal spinous processes undergoing autolytic debridement.

Dressings Used for Packing

✓ Dead space occurs when enough tissue is lost from a wound to leave a cavity where tissue should remain. The presence of dead space in a wound or surgical site provides the potential of seroma or hematoma formation.

♥ In either case, infection is a more common sequela than when the entire wound or surgical area can be closed. In some cases this is simply not possible and dead space remains.

✓ Gauze is the most commonly used dressing to fill dead space.

🖐 Roll gauze is preferred in order to have a contiguous dressing thereby minimizing the chance of leaving foreign material in the depths of the dead space. The gauze is unrolled and pushed into the defect until the defect is filled (Figure 1-4). If the defect is large and requires more than one roll, the end of the first roll is tied to the beginning of the next roll and so on. In this fashion, only one end of the gauze needs to be pulled until all of the gauze is removed.

✓ Woven gauze is preferred because it is stronger than non-woven gauze and is less likely to tear.

💣 The gauze should be moistened prior to application and kept moist to minimize drying of the wound and reduce the pain associated with removing the packing.

♥ Antimicrobial gauze such as Kerlix A.M.D. provides the benefit of reducing bacterial load while also filling the dead space.

♥ Any type of woven gauze will provide physical debridement and as long as it is pre-moistened will minimize trauma to the surrounding tissue. Specific dressing types will be described in more detail in Section 6.

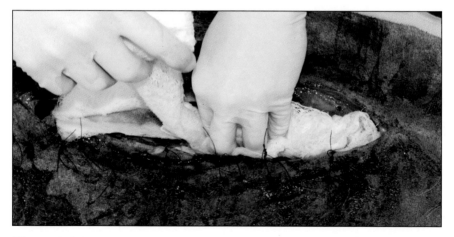

Figure 1-4 Dorsal spinous process wound being packed with saline moistened antimicrobial roll gauze (Kerlix A.M.D.™ Tyco Healthcare/Kendall).

Dressings Used for Absorption

✓ One of the more common uses for dressings is absorption. In this case, the dressing is used to contain drainage and exudate. Cotton is one of the better known dressings used for this purpose based upon its natural absorbency. It is available in many forms and from many different companies. Roll cotton is commonly available and is probably the most cost efficient of the different forms of cotton (Figure 1-5).

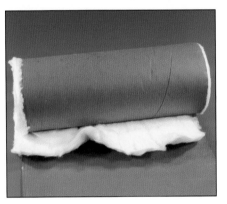

Figure 1-5 Roll cotton.

Products like Gamgee and Combine Cotton have a cotton layer covered by a non-adherent fabric (Figure 1-6). These dressings actually were described in 1880 by a doctor named Joseph Samson Gamgee, who wrote a paper describing use of bleached cotton pads covered with fine bleached cotton netting used by nurserymen to protect their plants from birds. These products now come in large rolls that are cut into smaller lengths for the specific need. Cotton also comes in sheets that can be layered and used similarly to other types of cotton (Figure 1-7).

Synthetic materials such as ABD pads (Tyco Healthcare/Kendall) are also available for absorption (Figure 1-8). In most cases, a gelatin-like material is encased between a non-porous plastic sheet and a non-adherent fabric. The non-adherent fabric layer is placed against the wound, allowing exudate to pass into the absorptive component, but stopping exudate from going back to the wound surface. The non-porous plastic layer stops exudate from penetrating from within and other fluids from penetrating from the outside. Disposable diapers work in much the same fashion and can be sterilized if necessary. Diapers often work better than the larger pads due to their size and conformability.

✋ It is important to use the appropriate dressing against the wound surface that will allow an appropriate amount of exudate to remain at the wound surface, yet allow excess exudate to be absorbed into the absorptive layer. This will be covered more in the section on Dressings Used for Moisture.

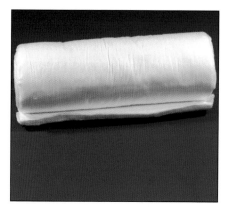

Figure 1-6 Combine cotton.

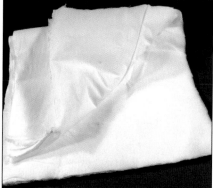

Figure 1-7 Sheet cotton.

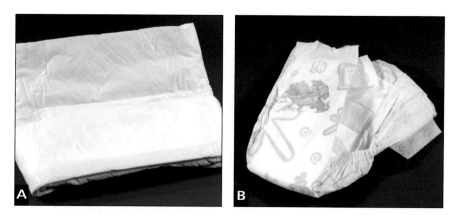

Figure 1-8 Absorbent secondary dressings. **A.** ABD™ Pad (Tyco Healthcare/Kendall), **B.** Disposable diaper.

Dressings Used for Compression

✓ Compression dressings are used to reduce or prevent swelling. In most cases, the various types of cotton described in the previous section are used under a pressure wrap such as roll gauze and an elastic bandage (Figure 1-9).

💣 It is important to achieve even pressure under the pressure wraps, or pressure sores may result. For this reason, the author prefers Combine cotton or sheet cotton for compression bandages.

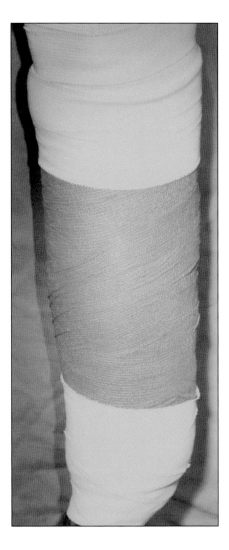

Figure 1-9 Compression bandage.

Dressings Used for Support

✓ Support dressings are essentially identical to compression dressings.

💣※ It is important to recognize that unless some type of external coaptation such as a splint is used, little benefit is gained with a support bandage in an adult horse (Figure 1-10).

⊙ For more information of splinting see Methods of Dressing Application at the end of this section.

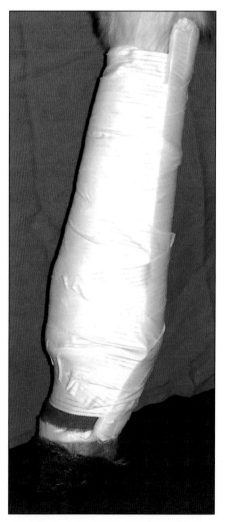

Figure 1-10 Support bandage with PVC pipe splint.

Dressings Used for Protection

✓ Protective dressings can be used to protect from both trauma and contamination. The dressings can be very thin and simple, or identical to compression dressings. Neonatal foals with flexural deformities can be protected with very light dressings, the goal being to protect the skin from abrasions. Heavy wraps in these cases will often exacerbate the flexural deformity.

🖐 One of the author's favorite dressings for protecting foals with flexural laxity is a tube sock (Figure 1-11). If more protection is necessary, a compression dressing can be used.

♥ Antimicrobial dressings like Kerlix A.M.D. have been designed to protect wounds from bacterial penetration, thereby reducing the likelihood of bacterial infection.

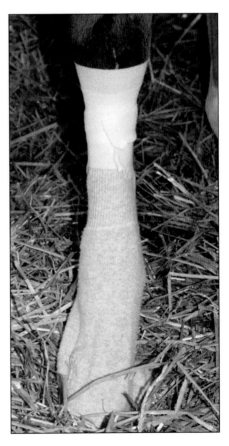

Figure 1-11 Tube sock on a foal with a flexural deformity.

13

Dressings Used for Moisture

✓ Dressings have become increasingly important in maintaining the proper moisture balance at the wound site (Figure 1-12).

♥ Optimal wound healing occurs when an appropriate moisture level is maintained at the wound bed.

☞ If a wound produces excess exudate, the appropriate dressing should allow exudate to move through the dressing into the absorbent layer of the bandage.

☞ If the wound is dry, the appropriate dressing will keep the wound exudate in contact with the wound bed.

✋ There can be a fine line between a wound that is too dry and a wound that is too moist. These dressings will be covered in more detail in Section 6.

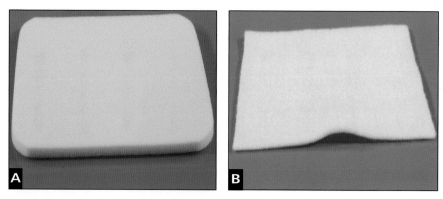

Figure 1-12 Pictures of occlusive dressings used for moisture retention. **A.** Semi-occlusive foam dressing, **B.** Calcium alginate dressing.

Methods of Dressing Application

♥ When a wound is present, an appropriate wound-care dressing should maintain the appropriate moisture balance and be held in place by roll gauze.

♥ When protection from bacteria is critical, it is beneficial to use antimicrobial roll gauze such as Kerlix A.M.D.™ to prevent bacterial penetration.

♥ If excess exudate is present, some type of absorbent dressing like cotton should be applied next.

♥ If there is too little exudate or the wound is dry, a plastic barrier may be used to maintain the moisture balance.

✔ Roll gauze should be applied over the cotton to provide even pressure. Elastic wraps should be placed over the roll gauze, again making sure to provide even pressure.

✔ When there is no wound, the first two layers can be omitted.

🖐 It has often been stated that the direction of rotation of the bandage material is important in order to reduce bandage complications. As far as the author knows, there is no evidence that rotation direction makes any difference on the other hand, even pressure and a good compressive layer (cotton) is very important.

🖐 However, it is important to recognize that some owners will expect the practitioner to place the dressing in a specific rotational direction so that if the bandage were to come undone, it would trail to the outside of the leg. Simply put, the dressing should be placed from medial to lateral, front to back (Figure 1-13).

⊙ Refer to CD for videos on dressing placement.

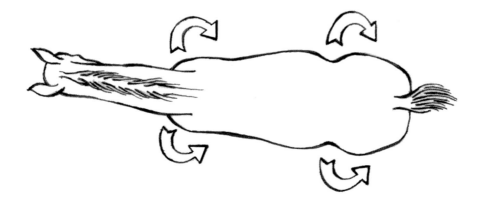

Figure 1-13 Drawing of horse from above showing direction of dressing rotation for the legs.

Splint Application

✓ There are many different types of splints available, including both commercial and "home made" varieties.

✓ The most commonly used commercial splint is the "Kimzey Splint." (Kimzey Welding Works) It is an aluminum splint that has a cradle for the foot and a bar that proceeds proximally on the dorsal surface (Figure 1-14). The splint comes in a standard size that extends from the ground to just below the carpus or hock. For the forelimb, an extension is available to extend the splint to the elbow. There are three different foot-cradle sizes available for small, medium and large sized feet. The splint incorporates nylon straps with velcro to fasten the splint to the leg and is valuable for almost any lower leg injury.

⊙ See video on CD for application of a Kimzey splint.

⬤ For fractures, the Kimzey splint should only be used if the fracture is in the distal portion of the metacarpus/metatarsus or distal on the leg.

✋ The main drawback is the cost of the splint. The author recommends charging a usage fee every time the splint is used, and requiring a deposit for the entire value of the splint if the horse owner is going to take the splint out of the practice. This will allow the practitioner to constantly upgrade the splint and replace it if it is not returned.

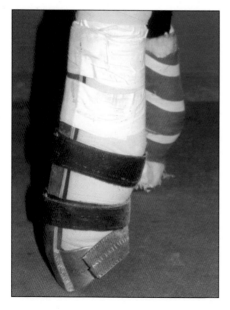

Figure 1-14 Picture of a horse in a Kimzey splint.

✓ Other materials that are commonly used for splints include polyvinylchloride pipe (PVC), wood, and casting material.

♥ These materials have the positive characteristics of being relatively cheap, and generally quite accessible.

☞ The author's recommendation is to keep some PVC pipe cut into 4-6 foot lengths, and 3-4 inch widths. Begin with a 6-to-8-inch diameter pipe that has a wall thickness of at least 1/4 inch (Figure 1-15). Cut the pipes into approximately 6-foot lengths with some type of saw. Use an electric hand-saw to cut the pipe longitudinally into strips that are 3 or 4 inches wide. File off the rough edges, and keep the precut lengths available for making a splint. If a horse needs a splint, cut the strips to the appropriate length with a saw and file the edges. The splints can be bent with a propane torch to make almost any desired configuration (Figure 1-16). The ends of the splints can be covered with cotton that is secured by tape to reduce the chance of pressure sores. PVC pipe splints have a built-in radius that will provide increased stability in two planes.

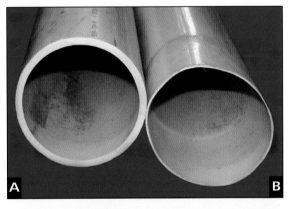

Figure 1-15 PVC pipe.
A. Supply with thick wall,
B. Drain with thin wall.

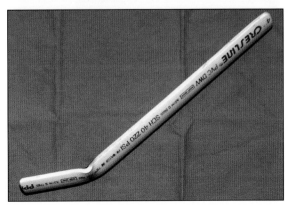

Figure 1-16 Cut and bent PVC pipe.

✓ Wooden splints can be made from any available wood type.

☞ It is generally beneficial to use two wooden splints at 90° from each other to provide the greatest stability. Two flat boards will provide better stability than two round boards (Figure 1-17).

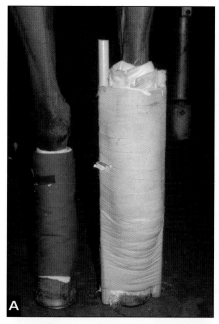
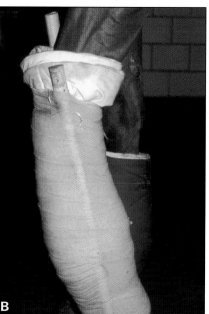

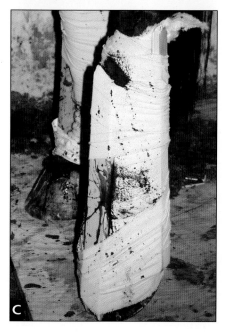

Figure 1-17 Wood splints. **A.** Dorsal view, **B.** Lateral view Improperly placed splints, **C.** Properly placed splints.

✓ Splints can also be made from cast material.

🖙 Generally a bandage is placed on the affected limb, then a roll of cast material is placed in water and unrolled on the front or back of the limb, but not around the limb (Figure 1-18). This is allowed to dry, and incorporated into the bandage. These allow more perfect form fitting than do any of the other splints, but they are generally more expensive to apply.

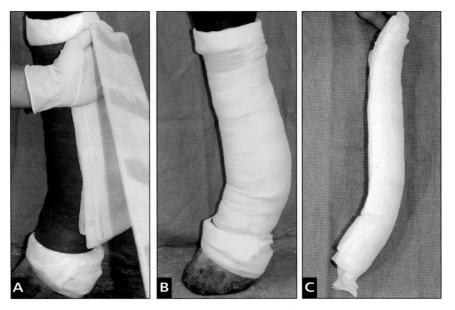

Figure 1-18 Cast material on the palmar aspect of a bandage. **A.** Applying cast material over pressure bandage, **B.** Finished splint with elastic bandage wrapped over the splint and the bandage, **C.** Cast material after curing.

💣 Any splint that is used should be applied over a good bandage and fixed in place with 2-3 inch non-elastic tape. It is best if the splint does not extend past the end of the support bandage unless an extended splint is used to support an upper limb fracture. If the splint does extend past the support bandage, the ends should be covered with cotton to reduce the chance of pressure sores.

Emergency Transport

🖙 Most horses with fractures need to be referred to a facility that can deal with the challenges of fracture repair.

💣 The objective of first aid in this instance is to minimize continuing trauma to the leg during transport. For a successful outcome, it is highly desirable to maintain the integrity of the surrounding soft tissue, and prevent the fracture from becoming open.

☝ If a fracture is suspected, it is usually prudent to place a bandage and a splint on the leg prior to radiographing or other manipulations. The type of splint and application of the splint will vary with the location of the fracture.

✋ A general rule of thumb is that the splint should immobilize the joint proximal and distal to the fracture. This is often not feasible in the horse, but should be accomplished if at all possible.

☝ For fractures occurring between the third phalanx and mid metacarpus/metatarsus, a splint should extend from the ground to the carpus or tarsus (Figure 1-19).

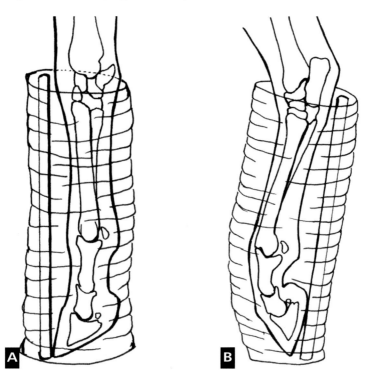

Figure 1-19 Drawing of distal leg splint. **A.** Forelimb, **B.** Hindlimb.

☝ For fractures occurring between the mid metacarpus and the distal radius, the splint should extend from below the fetlock to the point of the elbow (Figure 1-20).

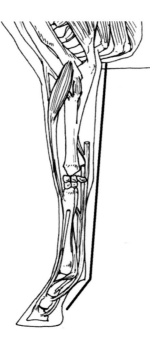

Figure 1-20 Splint extending from below fetlock to elbow.

For fractures occurring above the distal portion of the radius, a lateral splint should be applied to the withers (Figure 1-21). Fractures of the mid-metatarsus to the distal tibia can be immobilized with a similar lateral splint (Figure 1-22).

Fractures of the humerus and the femur can not be immobilized with external coaptation.

It is very important to remember that the splint and/or bandage should not end at the fracture. This only serves to add increased weight and instability to the lower leg, which will often lead to more severe injury to the affected bone and adjacent soft tissue.

When transporting an animal with a fracture, it is important to load and confine them in a trailer, giving them the best chance to support themselves without further injury.

Generally it is best to load the horses with the fractured leg facing the back of the trailer. If the driver has to "hit the brakes," the horse will be able to use its good legs for support during the rapid deceleration. The horse should also be confined as much as possible to allow the horse to support itself with its body when the trailer is turning.

Do not turn the horse loose in the trailer to find its own comfortable position.

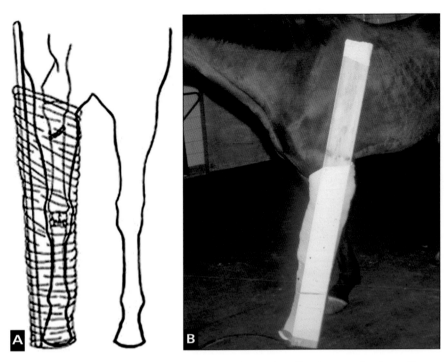

Figure 1-21 Spica splint. **A.** Drawing of spica splint, **B.** Picture of spica splint.

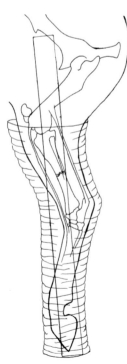

Figure 1-22 Drawing of hind-limb spica type splint.

Summary

✓ There are many dressing choices available to the veterinarian. Most of these dressings will be covered in complete detail in Section 6, Second Intention Healing.

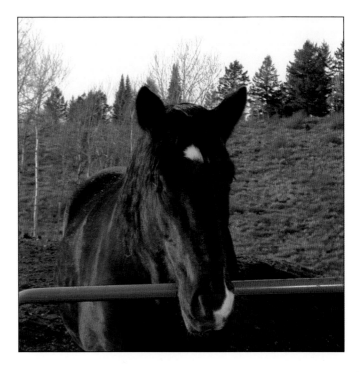

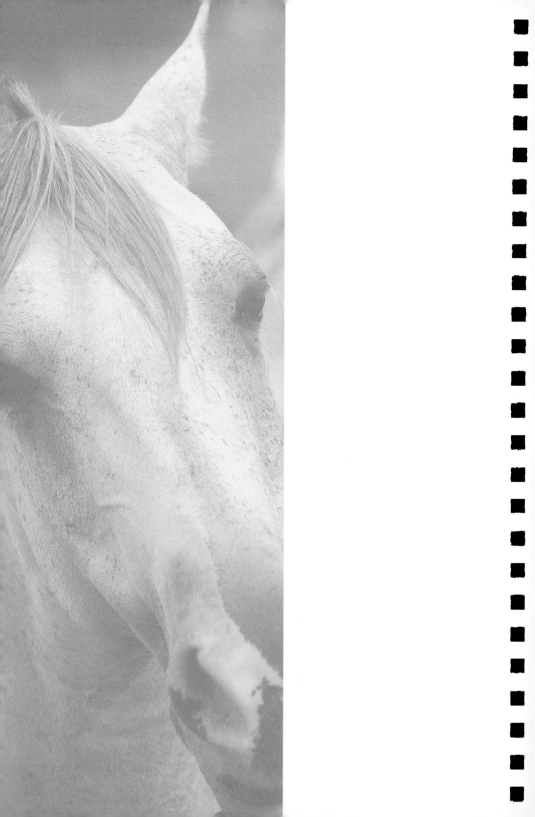

Section 2

Wound Preparation, Cleaning, and Debridement

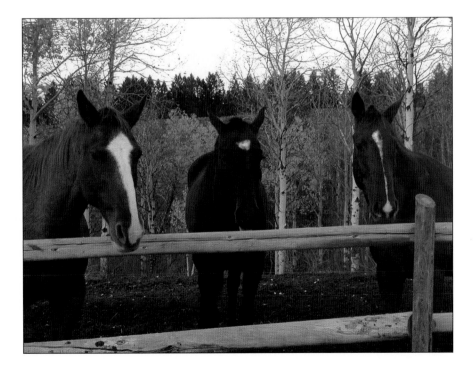

This section will help the practitioner to prepare a wound for examination, choose between multiple cleaning agents and techniques, and appropriately debride a wound.

✓ Lacerations come in all types and varieties. Horses may be presented with anything from simple abrasions, to lacerations that involve tendons, joints, major vessels and nerves as well as a host of other important structures.

💣 Due to this wide variance, it is of utmost importance that each patient receives a thorough physical examination to determine the extent of the problem as well as to determine the systemic status of the patient.

💣 If a major vessel has been severed it is easy for the horse to lose a substantial amount of blood, however clients will frequently overestimate the amount of blood lost.

🔑 After the initial physical examination to determine the systemic status of the animal, it is time to closely examine the affected area.

🔑 This may require some type of sedation and/or local anesthesia. You must remember that if a horse has lost a significant amount of blood, or is severely dehydrated, some sedatives (acepromazine, xylazine, and detomidine) can cause hypotension and circulatory collapse.

✓ It may be beneficial in these animals to use other agents such as local anesthetic or manual restraint (twitch, etc.) for the examination of the laceration or wound.

✓ Tetanus vaccination status should be determined prior to examination and a booster given if necessary.

Wound Preparation

♥ With most lacerations it is helpful to clip the hair surrounding the laceration prior to exploration. In one horse with a distal antebrachium laceration where the wound was not clipped, a veterinarian missed two small puncture wounds into the carpal joint (Figure 2-1). These wounds were by far the most serious and would have probably led to a septic arthritis.

🔑 The author uses a sterile water-soluble lubricating gel (for example, K-Y jelly) to fill the wound prior to clipping in order to prevent contamination with hair. The gel is placed in the wound by smearing the gel using a gloved hand (Figure 2-2). If the gel is

Figure 2-1 A horse with antebrachial and carpal wounds.

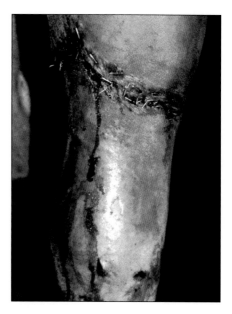

just squeezed into the wound it will often fall out before the clipping begins. The clipped hair will stick to the lubricant instead of the wound bed. Once the surrounding hair has been clipped, the lubricant can be rinsed out with sterile saline, scrub solution, or water if necessary.

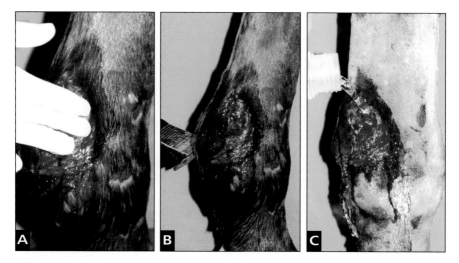

Figure 2-2 Horse with distal cannon wound. **A.** Sterile gel in wound prior to clipping, **B.** Clipping hair around wound, **C.** Rinsing gel and trapped hair from wound.

Wound Infection

✓ Most wounds will contain bacteria that come from either the animal itself or the environment.

♥ There are three main categories that are generally described when dealing with wound bacteria. **Wound contamination** is defined as the presence of bacteria that are not replicating within the wound. **Wound colonization** is defined as the presence of bacteria that are replicating but not causing trauma to the animal. These bacteria may actually be beneficial to the animal by reducing the adherence of pathogenic bacteria to the wound bed. For instance in humans the presence of *Corynebacteria sp.*, coagulase negative staphylococci, and viridans streptococci have been shown to actually accelerate healing. **Wound infection** is defined as the presence of bacteria that are replicating and causing trauma to the animal.

💣 The development of wound infection is dependent on the dose of bacteria, the virulence of the bacteria, and host resistance. Consequently the infective dose does not need to be very high if the bacteria is very virulent or if the host resistance is low. Large volumes of necrotic tissue will also tip the balance in favor of the bacteria. Careful cleaning and debridement of the wound to reduce the bacterial load and the amount of necrotic tissue will be beneficial in reducing the likelihood of wound infection. Chronic wound infection will often result in fragile granulation tissue and weak collagen in disorganized patterns leading to low tensile strength and reduced wound contraction. Infection should be considered in any wound that fails to heal despite providing the best possible wound-healing environment.

♥ Diagnosis of wound infection should be made clinically by assessing the local and systemic inflammatory response. Evidence of infection will include periwound cellulitis, erythema, swelling, and increased local temperature (Figure 2-3). Increased exudate with or without odor is often present.

🔑 Covert infection may have less obvious clinical signs and may include loss of granulation tissue or a change in the character of granulation tissue to more edematous, pale gray or deep maroon in color, and tissue that is more friable.

✓ Microbiological means of assessing bacterial load includes quantitative and qualitative bacteriology. Quantitative bacteriology will determine the amount of bacterial load present in a wound. It is generally accepted that bacterial loads of greater than 10^5 organisms per gram of tissue will negatively affect wound healing.

Figure 2-3 Picture of horse with longstanding infection.

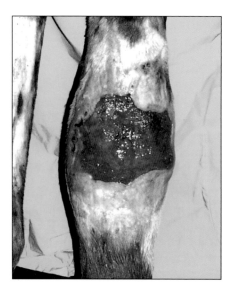

🖐 The addition of foreign material including; osteomyelitis, necrotic tissue, orthopedic implants, or suture material, will reduce the amount of bacteria necessary for an infection to 10^4 organisms per gram of tissue.

♥ Consequently foreign-body removal is critical in the quest for rapid and cosmetic wound healing.

✓ Quantitative bacteriology is rarely performed and should only be used as an adjunct to a complete clinical examination. Qualitative bacteriology will determine the particular species of organisms present in the wound. Different types of bacteria will have distinct virulence patterns, and affect the tissue differently. Specific bacteria will also require particular treatment modalities.

♥ Qualitative bacteriology along with sensitivity testing is probably the most useful technique in determining the appropriate treatment regimen.

Wound Cleaning Agents

🖐 One of the most important steps in wound healing is proper cleaning and thorough exploration of the wound. As described in the previous case in the wound preparation section, it is important to clean the entire area to make sure no small, but significant, wounds or foreign materials are present.

💣 *Cross contamination of the wound should be avoided in all cases.*

When dealing with an open synovial structure, strict aseptic technique should be used including sterile gloves and sterilized gauze. In other areas only clean gloves are required.

✔ Many different substances have been used to clean wounds prior to wound exploration and treatment.

💣 It is important to remember that the use of almost all wound-cleansing agents will cause trauma to the wound bed either by chemical means, mechanical means or a combination of both.

✔ Chemical trauma can result in cellular toxicity when the cleaning agents are not biocompatible. Mechanical trauma occurs when mechanical forces such as scrubbing or high pressure, are used.

♥ Therefore, the benefits of a clean wound must be weighed against the trauma that the agent will cause.

Simply put, the practitioner must determine if the cleaning agent will eventually speed up or retard wound healing. When choosing wound cleansing agents, a simple rule of thumb is "Don't do to a wound what you wouldn't do to your own eye."

Scrubbing

✔ Wound-cleansing activity can be enhanced with the addition of scrubbing devices such as woven or non-woven gauze (Figure 2-4). (See Section 1 on Dressings.) It is important to remember that mechanical trauma will ensue with the use of scrubbing devices.

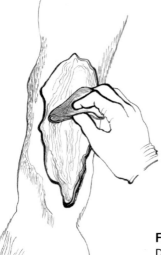

Figure 2-4
Drawing showing gauze debridement.

🔑 Woven gauze is more effective in removing tissue than non-woven gauze, but will create more tissue trauma when used. As always, it is important to balance the negative effect of mechanical trauma to the cells with the benefit of reducing foreign material at the wound site.

🔑 The practitioner should use the minimal amount of force necessary to remove the foreign material. Other cleansing agents or debridement techniques, not increased force, should be used if the initial attempt at removing foreign material is not successful.

Lavage

✓ Irrigation force is another important factor to consider when performing wound irrigation, regardless of the fluid used.

🔑 In general, higher pressures will be more effective in reducing bacterial numbers than lower pressures, but will be more traumatic to tissue. High-pressure systems will cause increased dispersion of fluid along tissue planes. It is recommended that fluid pressure not exceed 15 pounds per square inch (psi) to reduce fluid dispersion. Shower tips have also been shown to reduce the amount of fluid dispersion when compared to single-lumen tips. To achieve low-pressure lavage, 16 gauge needle holes can be placed in the top of a saline bottle (Figure 2-5).

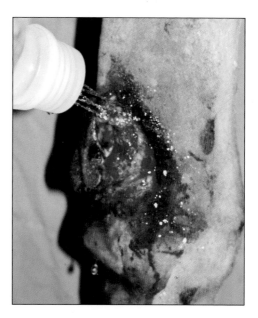

Figure 2-5
Saline bottle with holes in top being used for lavage.

Rodeheaver has shown that both the size of the syringe and the size of the needle used will determine the pressure of the fluid stream produced. When using a 35-ml syringe the pressures generated with a 25, 21, and 19-gauge needle are 4, 6, and 8, psi respectively. When using a 19-gauge needle with a 6, 12, and 35-ml syringe, pressures of 30, 20, and 8 psi are reached respectively (Figure 2-6). Many devices are currently available for fluid irrigation, some of which are battery powered that may allow the practitioner more latitude when performing wound irrigation. It is important to remember that more pressure is better only to a level of about 15-psi.

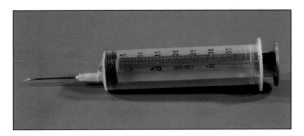

Figure 2-6 A 35-ml syringe with 19 GA needle.

Saline

✓ Normal or isotonic saline (0.9% NaCl) is a very effective wound-cleaning agent. In many situations with mildly contaminated wounds, saline is the agent of choice. Isotonic saline provides a fluid medium that will neither cause cells to swell like plain water will, nor crenate cells like hypertonic solutions will. Sterile saline should be used around synovial structures.

✓ Adding two teaspoons of salt to one liter of boiling water can make an acceptable lavage solution. Tap water can be used in grossly contaminated wounds, but saline is better when there is minimal contamination or wound healing is already advanced.

Antiseptic Agents

✓ Antiseptic agents are used for both skin preparation, and wound cleaning and lavage. Only those uses for wound cleaning and lavage will be discussed in this section.

☞ When treating wounds it is imperative to reduce the level of contamination to allow wound healing to proceed with the least amount of interference. While wound healing can occur with high numbers of bacteria, it is generally thought that it will occur faster and more cosmetically if bacterial numbers can be reduced.

✋ It is impossible to completely eliminate bacteria from a wound. If a wound is grossly contaminated, it is an important step to reduce the level of contamination with respect to foreign material and bacterial load.

☞ While it may seem more important to reduce the contamination than to worry about the cytotoxicity of the cleansing agent, it is important to use the least cytotoxic cleansing agent that will still provide a reduction in bacterial numbers.

✋ Topical antiseptics will not reduce the bacterial load in wound tissue. Topical or systemic antibiotics are needed to achieve this effect. Antiseptics will damage all cells on contact and are therefore non-selective in their effect. Numerous studies have shown the ability of antiseptics to kill bacteria, however, most of these studies have been performed by placing the bacteria into the fluid antiseptic where direct contact between the bacteria and the antiseptic is possible. The presence of wound exudate and necrotic tissue will reduce or completely eliminate the effectiveness of the antiseptics. Fleming in 1919 stated that it was impossible to sterilize a wound with an antiseptic, and no controlled clinical study to date has been able to disprove this conclusion.

♥ In many cases the antiseptics have mistakenly been given the credit for reduction in bacterial numbers, when, in fact, wound debridement was responsible for the reduction of bacterial load.

✔ Some of the more common antiseptic agents will be discussed in this section. These agents should only be used on the skin surrounding the wound (Figure 2-7).

☞ Appropriate debridement should be employed to reduce the volume of necrotic debris and bacterial numbers.

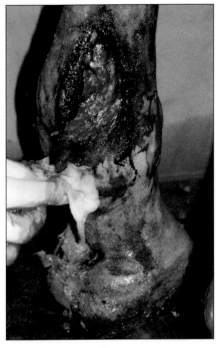

Figure 2-7 Use of povidone iodine scrub around but not in the wound.

Povidone-Iodine

✔ Povidone-iodine (Figure 2-8) has long been considered a gold standard, or a clinical standard of care to reduce bacterial numbers in wounds. Many studies have reported that povidone-iodine is effective in reducing the bacterial load and consequently improving wound healing. It is likely that the benefit achieved by povidone-iodine use is associated with the debridement that is occurring.

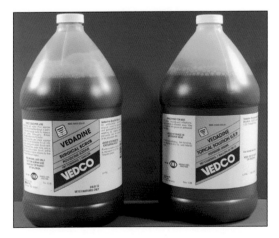

Figure 2-8
Picture of povidone iodine surgical scrub and solution.

🖐 In a study comparing the topical antibiotic silver sulfadiazine, povidone-iodine, or saline-soaked gauze, povidone-iodine was the least effective in reducing bacterial numbers in the wound.

✓ In another study saline alone was found to produce twice the amount of epithelial ingrowth of wounds treated with povidone iodine.

♥ Povidone iodine is best reserved for the periwound tissues.

Chlorhexidine

✓ Chlorhexidine (Figure 2-9) has been suggested to have a wide spectrum of activity, low systemic absorption and low systemic toxicity. It is reported to have a longer residual effect than povidone-iodine. Yet it is contraindicated for use around the cornea, the middle ear, and synovial structures.

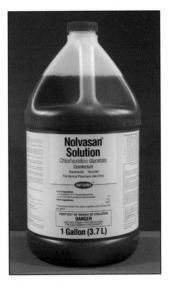

Figure 2-9 Chlorhexidine solution.

♥ As with povidone-iodine, deep infections will not be ablated with the use of chlorhexidine. If selected, the lowest possible concentration of chlorhexidine should be used to reduce cellular toxicity. Concentrations of 0.05% have been shown to be toxic to cells and bacteria.

🖐 Chlorhexidine is best reserved for the periwound tissues.

Hydrogen Peroxide

✓ Hydrogen peroxide (Figure 2-10) is most popular for its effervescent effects. This bubbling activity can be mistaken for antibacterial activity, which is actually quite low. The most likely benefit of hydrogen peroxide is that it might loosen and hasten the removal of necrotic debris in the wound.

🖐 The use of hydrogen peroxide should be discontinued once the necrotic tissue has been removed.

Acetic Acid

✓ Acetic Acid (vinegar) (Figure 2-11) has been described as having marked efficacy against Pseudomonas sp. and other aerobic gram-negative rods. The most likely reason for the proposed efficacy is the inability of these bacteria to tolerate the low pH environment caused by the acetic acid. The benefit of bacterial reduction must constantly be measured against the cellular toxicity. In many instances the low pH is not biocompatible with the wound tissue. Recommendations include a 15-min/day soak or compress. Acetic acid has also been recommended for odor control in some wound infections.

🖐 Use of acetic acid should be terminated once infection is under control.

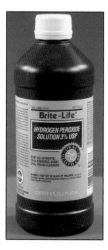

Figure 2-10
Hydrogen peroxide.

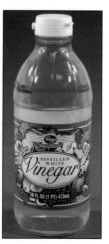

Figure 2-11
Vinegar (acetic acid).

Dakin's Solution

✓ Dakin's solution (Figure 2-12) is a 0.5% solution of sodium hypochlorite (bleach). The solution was first used on wounds during World War I. It acts as a chemical debriding agent in dissolving and removing necrotic tissue. As will be described in the debridement section, debridement of necrotic tissue is one of the best ways to decrease bacterial numbers.

🖐 Consequently Dakin's solution should only be used if necrotic tissue is present.

🖐 Many antiseptic agents have been used to reduce bacterial numbers. While they are very successful in in-vitro studies where bacteria are added to the antiseptic fluid, they are not successful when used to kill bacteria deep in wound tissue, yet they are toxic to cells. Many "magical" dilutions have been suggested to reduce cellular toxicity while also retaining antibacterial effects. While this may work in a test tube, it is not effective in a wound with all of the organic matter present.

🔑 In summary, antiseptics are very useful to clean the surface of a wound or the area surrounding a wound but they will not penetrate deeper into the wound to kill bacteria. Consequently, because of their cellular toxicity, they are probably not the best choice for wound cleaning and should not be used in clean wounds.

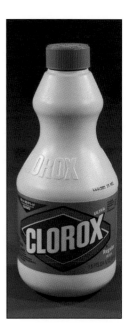

Figure 2-12 Bleach (for making Dakin's solution).

Topical Antibiotics

✓ Topical antibiotics have been very effective in reducing bacterial numbers in human burn patients. Commonly used systemic antibiotics should be avoided for topical use to reduce the chance of antimicrobial resistance.

🔑 A general rule of thumb is to use the topical antibiotics for two weeks or less, and to use an appropriate antibiotic for the bacteria that is found in the wound. A bacterial culture and sensitivity will best determine this.

Silver

✓ Silver (Figure 2-13) has been used in many formulations including: 0.5% silver nitrate solution, silver sulfadiazine cream, and silver impregnated dressings. Silver has been most commonly used in burn patients. The cream needs to be removed and replaced at least daily. The silver impregnated dressings have been designed to stop bacterial penetration but have not been made for use in open wounds to treat infections. In one study comparing burn wounds treated with collagenase combined with polymixin B and bacitracin versus silver sulfadiazine cream, the collagenase treated wounds healed more quickly. This underscores the concept that adequate debridement is more critical than topical antimicrobial therapy in wound healing. A recent study in horses comparing silver dressings, with and/or without secondary bandages, to povidone iodine showed no effect on the rate of epithelialization and wound contraction. Silver dressings without a secondary bandage were less likely to be associated with exuberant granulation tissue. More studies will have to be performed to determine the effectiveness of silver impregnated dressings in treating concurrent infections.

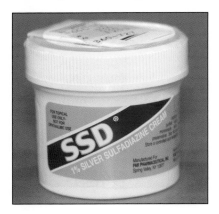

Figure 2-13 Silver sulfadiazine cream.

Nitrofurazone

✓ In one study, nitrofurazone (Figure 2-14) was compared to triple antibiotic ointment, povidone iodine, and silver sulfadiazine on the rate of wound healing. Nitrofurazone significantly retarded the healing rate.

☞ It has been shown that nitrofurazone in a concentration of 0.02% had a dose-dependent toxicity to cells, yet minimal effect against microorganisms. Other studies have shown similar effects, and it can not be recommended to use nitrofurazone on healing wounds.

☞ There are other products that are at least as effective in reducing bacterial numbers that are less cytotoxic to the wound bed.

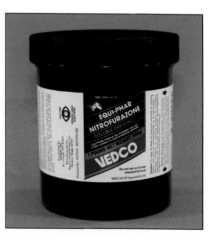

Figure 2-14 Nitrofurazone.

Triple Antibiotic: Neomycin/Polymixin B/Bacitracin

✓ Triple antibiotic ointment (Figure 2-15) has long been hailed as an effective agent for bacterial reduction and improved wound healing. Many studies have shown the benefit of triple antibiotic ointment when compared to other topical antiseptic or antimicrobial agents. The antibiotics work in a synergistic fashion, with the combination being more beneficial than any of the agents individually.

☞ More recent studies have shown that a moist wound-healing environment may be as beneficial as triple antibiotic in reducing bacterial numbers and more beneficial in stimulating wound healing.

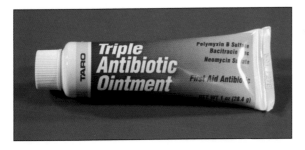

Figure 2-15 Triple antibiotic ointment.

Surfactant-Based Agents ⊙

✓ Wound cleansers with surfactants are designed to break down the surface tension and bond between foreign material and the normal host tissues. The strength of the surfactants are proportionate to the cleaning activity and the toxicity to cells.

☞ Consequently, cleansers that are the most effective in removing debris are also the most toxic. In one study using human fibroblasts, red blood cells, and white blood cells as test cells, Constant-Clens™ (Tyco Healthcare/Kendall) was the most biocompatible.

♥ In general surfactant-based wound cleansers are used in wounds with mild to moderate contamination and wound exudate (Figure 2-16). If minimal exudate is present, saline should be used.

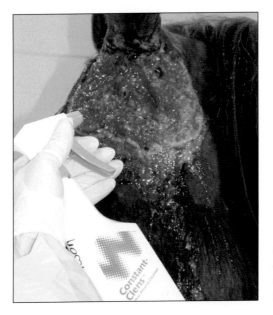

Figure 2-16 Surfactant based wound cleanser (Constant-Clens™ Tyco Healthcare/Kendall) in use in wounds.

☞ The author prefers to spray the wound with wound cleanser, then rinse the wound cleanser off with saline after allowing approximately one minute of contact time.

✓ Other detergents or soaps can be used to clean wounds. It has been proposed that 1/4 cup of liquid soap in 5L of warm water can be very effective in cleaning a wound. The main disadvantage of this method is that many soaps contain other additives that may be detrimental to the wound site.

✓ After the wound and surrounding area has been cleaned, the entire wound can be explored.

✋ It is important to assess all surrounding structures such as nerves, vessels, muscles, tendons, ligaments and bones to determine their involvement in the injury. (See Section 3 on Wound Exploration) If there is a large amount of bleeding from a large vessel, the vessel should be ligated at this time. The viability of the surrounding tissue should be evaluated, and compromised tissue should be debrided.

Wound Debridement

♥ Wound debridement centers around removing devitalized tissue, bacteria, and/or contaminants or foreign bodies. Presence of any of these agents can retard healing and inhibit the body from fighting off an infection.

☞ Wound debridement is one of the most effective and rapid methods of reducing bacterial contamination in a wound. It is important to realize that all types of debridement will both positively and negatively affect the wound bed, and consequently, wound healing. The best choice for debridement is one where the positive characteristics will outweigh the negative characteristics for the particular type of wound.

✓ There are many ways to provide wound debridement that will be broken into three main categories: mechanical, chemical, and natural debridement. Each of the main categories will be broken into more subcategories that will be discussed in this section.

Mechanical Methods

✓ Mechanical methods of debridement require some type of active physical contact with the wound bed by using some instrument or product that is not normally found in the wound. The most common mechanical methods include sharp and physical debridement.

Sharp Debridement

✓ Sharp debridement occurs when a means of cutting such as a scalpel, scissors, or laser is used to remove devitalized tissue (Figure 2-17). This is one of the most widely used forms of debridement.

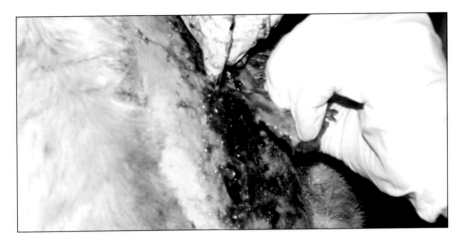

Figure 2-17 Sharp debridement post radiation therapy.

☞ Sharp debridement is the least traumatic of the mechanical methods, with the scalpel blade being the least traumatic of these modalities. Sharp debridement is a very definitive method in that once the tissues have been cut off, there is no turning back. Accurate debridement requires a good understanding of tissue viability since aggressive debridement can lead to a larger wound than necessary.

✋ It is generally best to be conservative when using sharp debridement. It is possible to reassess the viability of the tissues involved sequentially and remove a smaller amount of tissue each time. Using a conservative approach will maximize tissue remaining for wound healing.

☞ Large devitalized tissue flaps, large area of necrosis, or extremely contaminated wounds are best treated with sharp debridement or when quick debridement is necessary. It may be necessary to provide some type of anesthesia prior to performing sharp debridement, making the overall procedure more expensive.

Physical Debridement

✓ Physical debridement occurs when devitalized tissue is removed by physical forces other than those described in the sharp debridement section.

♥ It is generally cost effective and simple to perform. In many cases, this is performed with woven gauze that is "scrubbed" over the wound surface (see Figure 1-2).

✋ The practitioner must remember that this is a very traumatic modality and should be used sparingly. Excess pressure will not be beneficial to the wound-healing process. This technique is most useful for relatively small quantities of devitalized tissue.

✓ "Wet-to-dry" or "dry-to-dry" dressings can be used for physical debridement.

💣 The concept is to always keep the gauze moist. In many instances, woven gauze is placed on the wound surface and allowed to dry. The dry gauze is then removed, taking the devitalized tissue with it. In many situations healthy but fragile fibroblasts and/or epithelial cells are removed at the same time. Wet-to-dry or dry-to-dry bandages can be useful for physical debridement, but they require constant vigilance to reduce the trauma to the fibroblasts and epithelial cells and surrounding normal tissue.

🔑 The dressings should always remain moist to minimize trauma to the wound bed. In general, physical debridement is best reserved for wounds that have gross contamination and areas of devitalized tissue that are not contiguous.

✓ Hydrotherapy is another technique that can be used for physical debridement. Many systems are available, but a 35cc syringe with a 19-gauge needle will provide a cost-effective method of performing hydrotherapy. Increased pressure beyond 15 psi is not helpful in the wound-healing process.

🔑 Physical debridement is generally considered to be non-selective and may damage normal tissue delaying wound-healing by continued wound trauma. It is also considered to be painful for the patient and should be used sparingly. Other types of debridement such as autolytic debridement will generally provide better results when less contamination is present.

Chemical Debridement

Chemicals

✓ Chemical debriding agents have been available for some time, but often the trauma to the rest of the wound bed is significant enough to overshadow the benefits of the chemicals. Dakin's solution is one of the most common currently used chemical debriding agents.

☞ The excessive trauma associated with chemical debridement often precludes its use.

Hypertonic Saline Dressings

✓ Hypertonic saline dressings have been designed for use on infected or heavily exuding wounds (Figure 2-18). The hypertonic saline works by osmotic action to desiccate the necrotic tissue and bacteria in a wound. Debridement is very effective in reducing the number of bacteria in the wound.

☞ The debridement is non-selective and must be carefully monitored to make sure the surrounding tissue is not damaged.

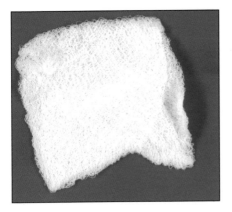

Figure 2-18 Hypertonic saline (Curasalt™ Tyco Healthcare/Kendall) dressing.

✋ Dressings should be changed every 24 to 48 hours at the onset of treatment, but can be left longer once the infection is under control. Hypertonic saline dressings work similarly to wet-to-dry dressings, but are more efficient and less traumatic to surrounding tissue.

♥ The author has used 20%, 10%, and 7.5% hypertonic saline

on woven gauze and has found the 20% hypertonic saline (Curasalt™- Tyco Healthcare/Kendall) to be the most effective. Loosely woven gauze dressings are the most efficient in debridement when combined with hypertonic saline.

🖐 These dressings should be discontinued once the wound has been effectively debrided.

Natural Methods

✓ Natural methods of debridement make use of naturally occurring substances to achieve debridement.

🔑 This is the most selective method of debridement but also requires the most patience.

Autolytic Debridement

♥ Autolytic debridement is achieved under semi-occlusive or occlusive dressings when the wound fluid is allowed to stay in contact with the wound bed (Figure 2-19). The body's own enzymes are used to soften the eschar and remove necrotic tissue.

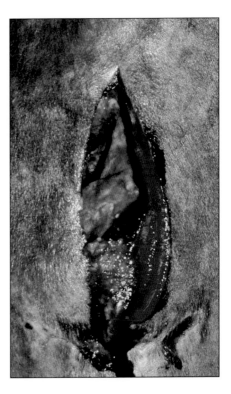

Figure 2-19 Autolytic debridement.

If a wound has become dry, it takes between 72 and 96 hours, depending upon the thickness of eschar and the size/location of the wound, for the autolytic debridement to begin. A moist environment allows better migration of neutrophils and macrophages than a dry wound environment. Neutrophils and macrophages phagocytize bacteria and debris while releasing enzymes to further promote debridement. Other enzymes in the wound fluid act to remove the devitalized tissue in a similar fashion. Chemotactic factors are released, stimulating the migration of more neutrophils and macrophages to phagocytize bacteria and debris. Autolytic debridement is very selective and only removes devitalized or diseased tissue, leaving healthy tissue intact to begin the healing process.

⌥ Autolytic debridement is considered a painless debridement, is usable on many surfaces, and is easy to perform.

✋ Large volumes of devitalized tissue would provide too large a task for autolytic debridement alone and should be debulked sharply, if possible, prior to occlusive dressing application.

✋ Autolytic debridement is not the best technique to use on heavily infected wounds, and clients should be warned to watch the wound for infection. It is not uncommon for wounds undergoing autolytic debridement to be associated with an anaerobic odor, even without the presence of infection.

Enzymatic Debridement

♥ Enzymes applied for enzymatic debridement are fast acting and selective to the tissues that need to be removed. Common enzymes are streptokinase/streptodornase, collagenase, DNAse/fibrinolysin, papain/urea, and trypsin. The enzymes attack the necrotic debris at different levels, liquefying the debris and allowing for easy removal. The normal tissue that surrounds the wound is left intact. Enzymatic debridement is best used on large wounds with mild to moderate amounts of necrotic debris.

⌥ The major deterrent to enzymatic debridement is the cost of the enzymes.

♥ In summary, there are many ways to debride a wound. The most effective choice should be made for each specific wound type. In most cases patience should be exercised so that only the devitalized tissue is removed. If the tissue viability is questionable it should be left and if necessary removed at a later time. Sharp and physical debridement techniques are the most common techniques used in veterinary medicine, but are not always the best method for debridement. Autolytic debridement is a very cost-effective method that is fairly easy to perform.

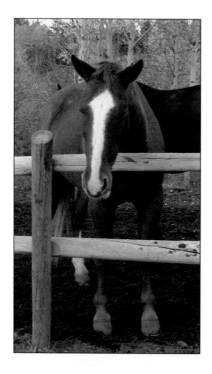

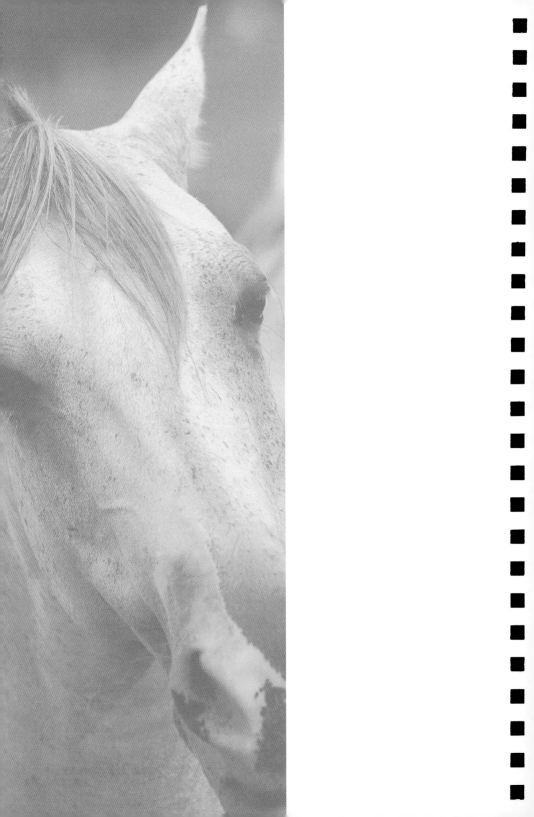

Section 3

Wound Exploration

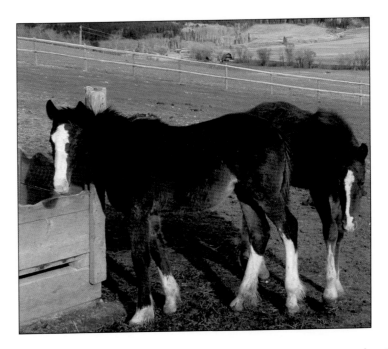

♥ This section will help the practitioner understand how to perform a complete wound exploration. Some of the anatomy that is commonly affected in equine wounds will be discussed. Keep in mind that a complete working understanding of anatomy is essential when performing wound exploration.

⚷ It is important to expertly assess all surrounding structures such as nerves, vessels, muscles, tendons, ligaments and bones to determine their involvement in the injury.

⚷ However, this section is not intended to be an all-inclusive anatomy lesson, so the reader should supplement this information with anatomy textbooks.

⬤ Before a thorough examination can be performed, the wound must be appropriately prepared. Wound preparation and cleaning are described in depth in the previous section. In all cases, the wound should be clipped prior to exploration. Many serious wounds have been overlooked because a practitioner failed to prepare and clean the affected area completely (Figures 3-1 and 3-2).

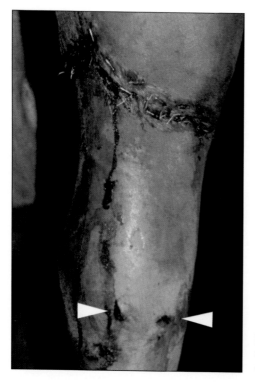

Figure 3-1 Picture showing horse with antebrachial and carpal wounds (arrows).

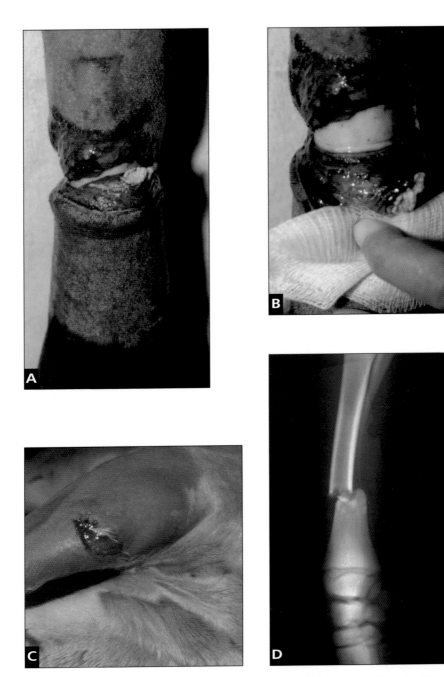

Figure 3-2 Horses with wounds with minimal superficial trauma, but significant deeper involvement. **A** and **B**: Wound caused by high tensile wire. **A**. Skin and extensor tendon laceration, **B**. Skin moved away to show grove in cannon bone caused by wire. **C** and **D**: Wound caused by a kick leading to a fractured radius. **C**. Right front leg with wound, **D**. Radiograph showing transverse radial fracture.

✋ If the setting is not conducive to proper preparation, the animal should be moved to a location that is more appropriate.

⚷ One of the author's greatest frustrations, is being presented with a horse that has a career-ending or life-threatening wound that was missed due to improper preparation. While the animal might have had a good prognosis from a practitioner's thorough preparation, cleaning and exploration, a poor prognosis resulted from insufficient technique. The old axiom holds true that many more things are missed for not looking than for not knowing.

✓ After the wound has been cleaned, it is time to perform a complete exploration.

✋ If the animal has not been sedated or local anesthesia has not been performed, this is generally a time when the animal will react. If the systemic status of the animal is acceptable, sedation will make the practitioner's job easier and will maximize the exploration.

⚷ If the animal is moving too much, the practitioner must do whatever is necessary to limit movement. Local anesthetic can be very useful in doing so.

💣 It is the practitioner's responsibility to do whatever it takes to provide the best circumstances for a complete and thorough exploration. It is not acceptable to settle for second best when it comes to wound exploration. A thorough exploration in some cases will only require the practitioner's hands and eyes. In other cases, the exploration will require adjunct diagnostic tools such as radiography and ultrasonography.

Head Wounds

✓ Head wounds can provide a diagnostic challenge, yet it is very important to understand the extent of the injury. Never assume that the wound is only superficial until a complete wound exploration has confirmed that.

♥ In one case, a horse had been spooked during a storm and was presented to the referring veterinarian the following day for a small wound between the ear and the eye. The wound was not clipped or explored. The horse was placed on antibiotics but did not improve. Eventually the wound was more thoroughly explored, and a tree branch approximately 3/4 inch in diameter and 4 inches long was found in the soft tissues behind the eye.

The horse lost the eye and was eventually euthanatized. Digital exploration and/or the use of ultrasound, may have led to the discovery of the stick, providing faster, more appropriate, treatment.

✓ Thorough exploration should rule out fractures (Figure 3-3), penetrations into the sinuses, lacerated salivary ducts (Figure 3-4), tongue lacerations, and injuries to the eyes.

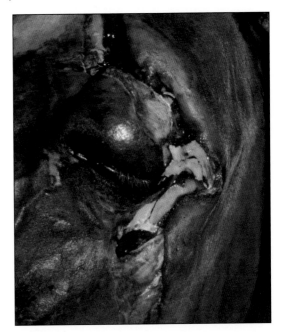

Figure 3-3 A severe head laceration involving the bony orbit and the eye.

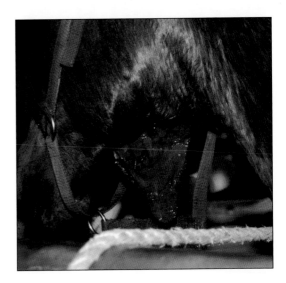

Figure 3-4 A horse with a throat latch laceration.

♥ One horse was presented with a history of having hit its head on a feeder after being spooked three days previously. The horse had very slight central nervous system abnormalities, and upon further evaluation, a fracture of the cranium was diagnosed.

✔ Radiographs, ultrasound, CT, and MRI all can provide useful information for head wounds. With complicated head trauma, a CT scan can be very helpful in diagnosing affected structures (Figure 3-5).

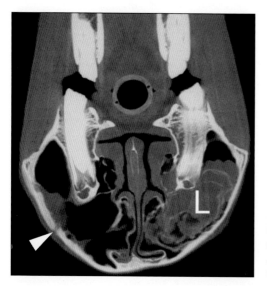

Figure 3-5 A CT scan of the maxillary sinus region of the head. Note the soft tissue filling of the left maxillary sinus (L), and the fracture of the right maxilla (arrow).

Neck and Back Wounds

☞ Neck wounds must be explored to determine the involvement of critical structures such as the jugular vein, carotid artery, trachea, and esophagus. Digital exploration is critical in determining the integrity of these structures.

✔ Endoscopy can be used to assess the involvement of the trachea and the esophagus. Ultrasound can be very useful in the neck region, but it can be complicated and challenging to evaluate.

✔ Back wounds should be examined for concurrent injury to the vertebrae and ribs. Fractures of the dorsal spinous processes should be identified at the time of injury to monitor for sequestrum formation.

✔ Digital exploration and radiographs are the most useful diagnostic techniques.

Chest Wounds

✓ Chest wounds might be superficial and involve only the superficial layers, or deep enough to enter the pleural cavity.

💣 You must be prepared for any eventuality when treating thoracic wounds.

🖐 Part of the thorough physical examination should include auscultation of the thorax.

🗝 After clipping and cleaning the wound, the wound should be digitally explored to identify an entry into the pleural cavity. In one case, the author heard a noise when the wound was being cleaned and debrided. Upon further evaluation, it was determined that the pectoral wound communicated with the thorax, and the noise was air being sucked into the pleural cavity upon inspiration (Figure 3-6).

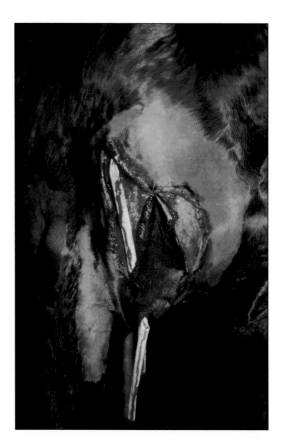

Figure 3-6 A horse with a pectoral wound.

✓ Careful examination of the ribs should be performed to rule out any fractures. If available, radiographs of the chest may help to rule out a concurrent pneumothorax (Figure 3-7).

💣 If thoracic involvement is suspected, the wound should be closed in multiple layers to decrease the likelihood of pneumothorax. If the facilities and equipment are available, a chest drain should be placed (Figure 3-8).

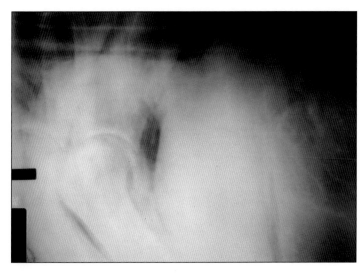

Figure 3-7 Radiograph of the horse in Figure 3-6 showing a pneumothorax.

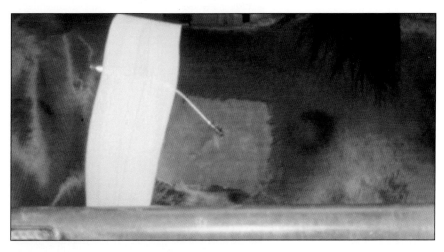

Figure 3-8 The horse in Figure 3-6 showing a chest tube in the right hemi-thorax.

Abdominal Wounds

✋ Wounds to the abdomen may penetrate into the peritoneal cavity. After the wound has been clipped and cleaned, the wound should be digitally explored using aseptic technique (Figure 3-9).

☞ There are often many fascial planes involved in abdominal lacerations, and a full exploration can be time consuming.

✋ Deep wounds may lead to evisceration or herniation, and should be wrapped until they can be adequately repaired.

💣 If a wound penetrates the peritoneum, there is always the possibility that the abdominal contents have been traumatized, which may worsen the prognosis significantly. In these cases, an abdominal exploration under general anesthesia should be suggested.

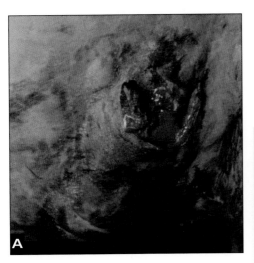

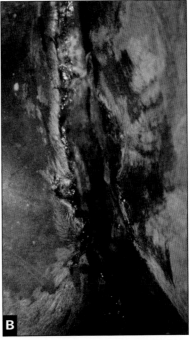

Figure 3-9 Horses with abdominal wounds. **A.** Laceration on the barrel of the abdomen, **B.** Flank laceration.

Leg Wounds

✓ There are many structures in the legs including bones, tendons, ligaments, nerves, and vessels. Consequently, wounds involving the legs can be simple or very complex, and should never be taken for granted.

☞ It is possible for the skin wound to look quite modest while the underlying structures are more severely involved (see Figure 3-2). The author has seen at least one horse with a palmar cannon bone laceration, where the superficial flexor tendon was noted to be intact immediately deep to the laceration. Upon further examination, the deep digital flexor tendon was completely transected. This case underscores the importance of a complete examination. The tendon was repaired, and the horse returned to athletic function.

✓ After the leg is clipped and the area cleaned, examination of the wound should be performed with the animal bearing weight and elevating the leg. It is generally helpful to move the leg through a range of motion to determine if more structures are involved.

☞ The leg should be stressed in the medial to lateral plane to rule out collateral ligament damage (Figure 3-10). Stressed radiographs may be required to rule out collateral ligament injury.

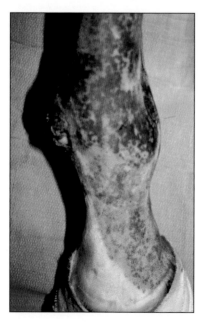

Figure 3-10 Lateral collateral ligament rupture.

♦ If involvement of a synovial structure is possible, it is critical to rule out penetration of the synovial membrane. Lacerations that involve synovial structures require immediate treatment to give the patient the best chance at recovery.

☞ In all cases, the best way to determine the involvement of a synovial structure begins with a good understanding of the underlying anatomy of the leg. It is important to understand the extent of the synovial pouches surrounding joints and tendon sheaths. It may be possible to determine the involvement of a synovial structure by palpation of the laceration and manipulation of the limb. If involvement cannot be confirmed with palpation and manipulation, it is possible to aseptically prepare a remote site (preferably one not involved with the laceration) and inject sterile saline into the synovial pouch to check for leakage at the laceration site (Figure 3-11). If the synovial structure is involved, there are many options for therapy, but all of them require aggressive and immediate action.

✍ If the practitioner is not confident about ruling out synovial involvement, the owners should be given the option of referral.

✔ Radiographs and ultrasound are useful techniques for assessing the integrity of bones and tendons or ligaments, respectively.

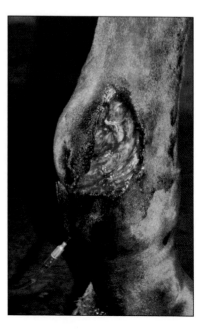

Figure 3-11 Injection of the digital tendon sheath to assess communication with a laceration.

Important Anatomical Considerations

✔ While there are many anatomic structures in the leg, the following table contains a list of anatomic structures that should be evaluated when faced with wounds in certain regions. This list is not all-inclusive and should be used as a minimum not a maximum.

Table 3-1
Anatomic Structures to be Evaluated

REGION	IMPORTANT STRUCTURES
Foot (Figure 3-12)	Coronary band
	Distal interphalangeal joint (Coffin joint)
	Third phalanx (Coffin bone)
	Navicular bursa
	Deep digital flexor tendon
	Digital arteries, veins, and nerves
Pastern (Figure 3-13)	Digital tendon sheath
	Proximal interphalangeal joint (Pastern joint)
	Collateral ligaments of the pastern joint
	Distal first phalanx
	Second phalanx
	Distal sesamoidian ligaments
	Deep digital flexor tendon
	Superficial digital flexor tendon
	Digital arteries, veins, and nerves
Fetlock (Figure 3-14)	Digital tendon sheath
	Metacarpal/Metatarsal phalangeal joint (Fetlock joint)
	Distal Metacarpus/Metatarsus III
	Proximal first phalanx (P1)
	Annular ligament
	Deep digital flexor tendon
	Superficial digital flexor tendon
	Proximal sesamoids
	Collateral ligaments of the fetlock joint
Cannon (Figure 3-15)	Digital tendon sheath
	Carpal tendon sheath
	Deep digital flexor tendon
	Superficial digital flexor tendon
	Suspensory ligament
	Metacarpus/Metatarsus III (Cannon bone)
	Metacarpus/Metatarsus II and IV (Splint bones)

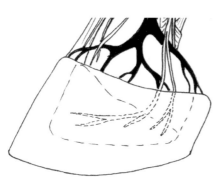

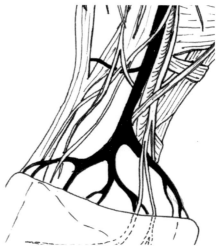

Figure 3-12 Drawing showing some of the anatomy of the foot region.

Figure 3-13 Some of the anatomy of the pastern region.

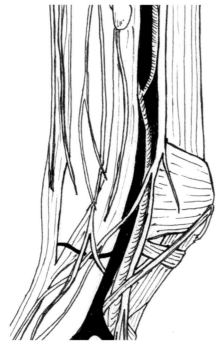

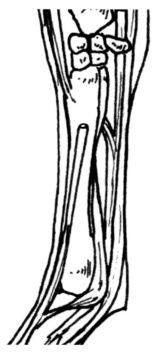

Figure 3-14 Drawing of some of the anatomy of the fetlock region.

Figure 3-15 Drawing of some of the anatomy of the cannon region.

Table 3-1 Continued

Region	Important Structures
Carpus (Figure 3-16)	Carpal joints
	Carpal bones
	Collateral ligaments of the carpal joints
	Carpal tendon sheath
Antebrachium (Figure 3-17)	Radius
	Ulna, especially olecranon
	Major muscle groups
	Radial nerve
Humerus, Shoulder, and Scapula (Figure 3-18)	Scapulo-humeral joint
	Humerus
	Scapula
	Bicepital bursa
	Bicepital tendon
Hock (Figure 3-19)	Tarsal joints
	Tarsal bones
	Distal tibia
	Collateral ligaments of the tarsal joints
	Deep digital flexor tendon
	Superficial digital flexor tendon
Tibia (Figure 3-20)	Tibia
	Fibula
	Gastrocnemius tendon
	Peroneus tertius tendon
Head	Calvarium
	Facial bones
	Sinuses
	Eye
	Tongue
	Teeth
	Salivary structures
Neck	Jugular vein
	Carotid artery
	Trachea
	Esophagus
	Vertebra
Thorax	Integrity of the thoracic wall
	Ribs
Abdomen	Integrity of the abdominal wall
Pelvis	Rectum
	Perineum
	Vulva
	Pelvis

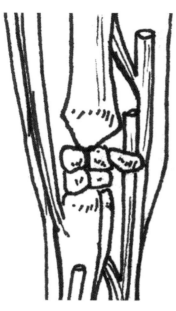

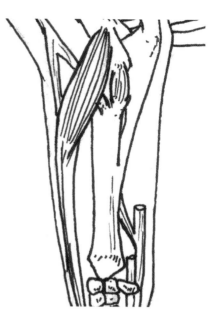

Figure 3-16 Drawing of some of the anatomy of the carpal region.

Figure 3-17 Some of the anatomy of the antebrachial region.

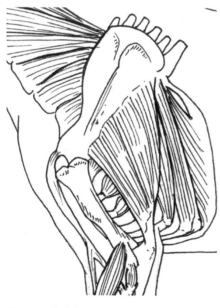

Figure 3-18 Some of the anatomy of the humeral, shoulder and scapular regions.

Figure 3-19 Drawing of some of the anatomy of the hock region.

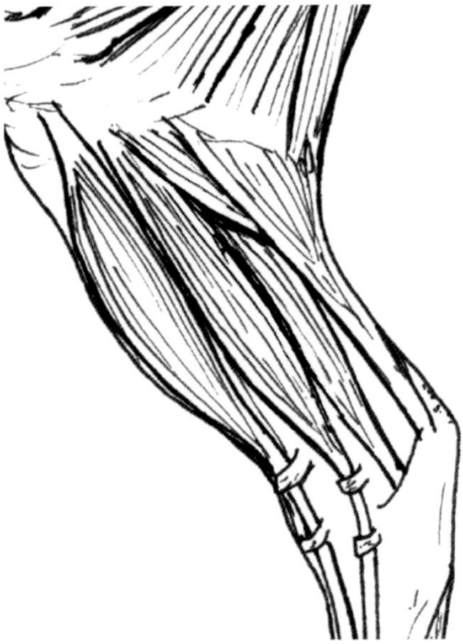

Figure 3-20 Drawing showing some of the anatomy of the tibial region.

Foreign Body Detection

✓ Foreign body detection is a very important part of wound care.

☞ The presence of a foreign body or foreign material reduces the number of bacteria necessary to establish an infection by one log, prolongs wound healing, and often results in a poor cosmetic outcome. Consequently, it is important to identify foreign material early in the wound-healing period.

✋ If a wound does not heal in the anticipated time frame, foreign material should be suspected until proven otherwise.

✓ There are many ways to identify foreign materials. They will be discussed from the most simple to the most complex.

Exploration

✓ Manual exploration is eventually used in all cases for finding foreign material. It can be used with any of the following techniques or as the sole technique.

✓ Manual exploration is the most cost-effective method available, requires the least sophisticated instrumentation, and can be performed anywhere.

♥ The most critical tool is a good understanding of pertinent anatomy. If the practitioner unfamiliar with a certain area, it will be hard to determine if there are any abnormalities.

✓ The least complicated method of manual exploration is to put on a pair of gloves (to avoid further contamination of the wound) and palpate the area (Figure 3-21). If possible, it is recommended to move the affected area around to make sure there are no occult pockets in the wound.

🖑 Aseptic technique should be used when the wounds are near synovial structures, the thorax, or the abdomen.

✓ Surgical exploration can be used when the wounds are too deep to explore manually, or are in areas where access is limited.

⚿ The more longstanding the wound, the more difficult manual exploration becomes.

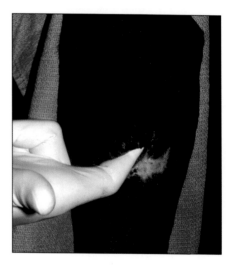

Figure 3-21 Palpating a wound at the dorsum of the carpus.

Ultrasound

✓ The advent of ultrasound has been a great asset in the search for radio-lucent foreign material (Figure 3-22).

⚿ It is very important to understand the principles of ultrasound and the anatomy of the area under examination. Without these understandings, it is possible to perceive almost anything as a foreign body, or to overlook a foreign-body entirely.

✓ In most cases, there is another side or limb of the horse to provide a comparison for normal examination. Don't hesitate to clip the contra-lateral side of the horse and practice scanning to understand what normal looks like.

⚿ Unless the area under examination is very thick, ultrasound is probably the best technique to use.

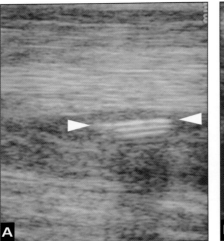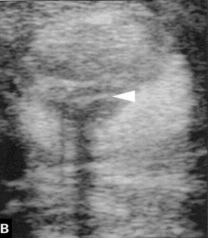

Figure 3-22 Ultrasound pictures at the level of the proximal cannon bone showing foreign material in the carpal canal. Note the shadowing under the foreign body (arrows). **A.** Longitudinal view, **B.** Cross section.

Plain Radiology

✓ Plain radiology is a very useful technique for finding metal or bone in a wound. (Figure 3-23)

☞ Two radiographs taken 90 degrees from each other (for example, lateral-medial and dorso-palmar) are necessary to localize the foreign body.

✓ A good three-dimensional understanding of the anatomy is helpful when using radiology.

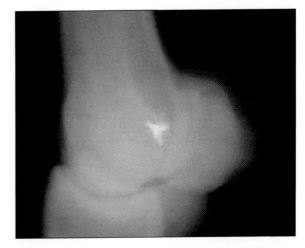

Figure 3-23 Radiograph with a fly overlying the sesamoid. The fly was actually in the cassette, not in leg.

Contrast Radiography

✓ Contrast radiography is valuable when a draining tract is present. The wound area is cleaned, and contrast material is injected into the wound cavity. If possible, a balloon catheter is used to maintain positive pressure of the contrast material and keep it in place for the radiograph. Filling defects will outline radio-lucent material (Figure 3-24).

☞ Two radiographic views will help the practitioner identify the location of the foreign material.

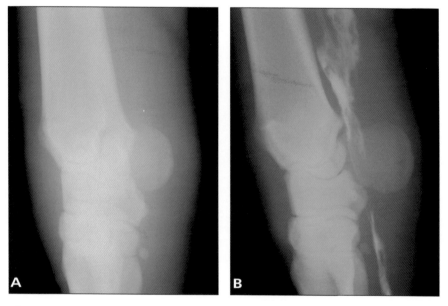

Figure 3-24 A radiographic contrast study in the same horse as Figure 3-22 showing wood foreign bodies. **A.** Standard radiograph showing no abnormalities, **B.** Contrast study of the carpal canal, note the filling defects, indicating foreign material.

Computed Tomography and Magnetic Resonance Imaging

✓ CT and MRI are great imaging modalities. Unfortunately, they are not widely available, and they are expensive. However, if an animal warrants the use of these modalities, and they are available, they will provide the best information available for foreign-body location.

☞ The main caveat is that they are currently only useful for the head, neck, and distal extremities.

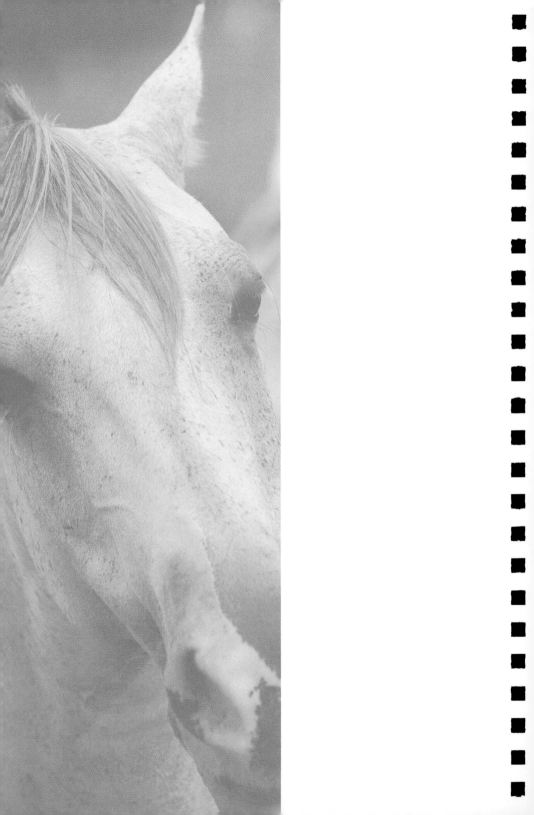

Section 4

Primary Wound Closure

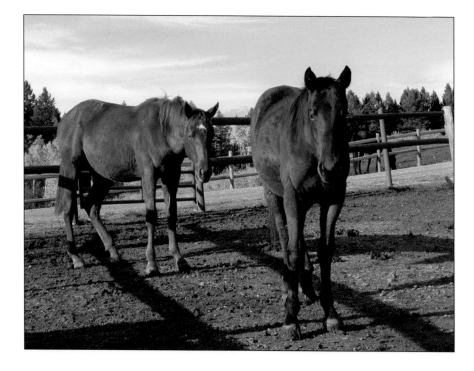

This section will help the practitioner to determine which wounds to close primarily, describe appropriate suture materials and patterns, and discuss wound immobilization.

☝ Primary wound closure is the preferred method for treating wounds. The end result is often more cosmetic, and is achieved with less time and effort than second-intention healing. Primary closure is most commonly performed with surgical incisions.

♥ In some cases with lacerations and wounds, primary-closure techniques can still be performed.

Appropriate Wounds for Primary Closure

☝ Primary wound closure is only appropriate in wounds that have adequate tissue to allow skin apposition with minimal tension.

☝ In addition to minimal tension, the wound must be free of gross contamination, bacterial infection, and foreign material.

☝ There should be minimal dead space left after closure of the wound (Figure 4-1).

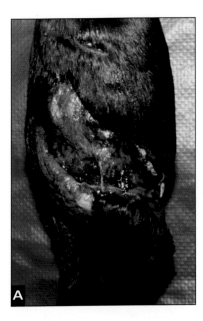

Figure 4-1
Carpal wound that underwent primary closure. **A.** Wound at presentation. **B.** Wound after debridement. **C.** Wound after primary closure. Note use of tension relieving and appositional sutures. **D.** Horse after surgery with cast on affected limb.

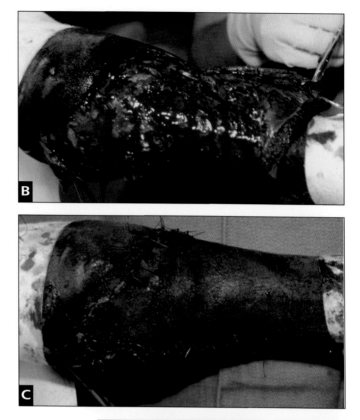

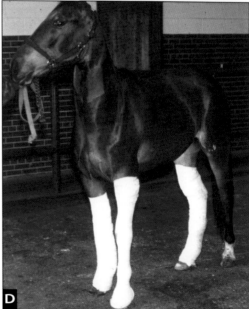

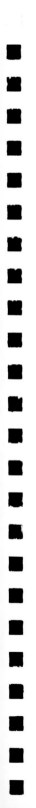

♥ There is no absolute standard for the amount of time after a wound has occurred that rules out primary wound closure. Rather the practitioner must examine the wound, identify all anatomic structures involved, and then determine if the wound has appropriate characteristics that would allow primary wound closure. Some wounds that are very fresh have too much debris and bacterial contamination for immediate closure while other wounds that are 24 hours old are very fresh and can be easily closed.

🖐 It is imperative to clip the hair around the wound, clean the area, and explore the wound thoroughly as explained in previous sections, before proceeding.

✓ The biggest contradiction to primary closure is that some wounds will dehisce in the post-operative period.

🔑 If this happens, it is important to re-examine the wound to check for infection, sequestration, or foreign material. After a thorough evaluation, the wound should be allowed to heal by second-intention healing.

✓ There are many techniques available for reducing dead space in a wound. Drains are the most commonly used method. Drains can either be passive or active.

🔑 Drain position is critical in providing the best drainage and reduction of dead space. Passive drains should be positioned so that the drain exits the wound at the most dependent area possible. Examples of passive drains are penrose drains and bandage drains (Figure 4-2). A passive drain should not exit at the proximal extent of the wound. Care must be taken to not include the drain in any of the layers of suture closure or drain removal will be difficult. Passive drains should be removed two to four days after placement. Active drains require some type of fenestrated rigid tubing and a vacuum device. An inexpensive vacuum device is a syringe with a three-way stopcock and a needle (Figure 4-3). Active drains are most commonly used in areas like the pleural cavity, peritoneal cavity, synovial structures, or very deep wounds. While active drains are very effective in the early stages, they can become plugged with fibrin or other debris, rendering them useless.

🖐 It is important to remember that ascending infections are possible whenever a drain is placed. When the drain is removed it is wise to submit the drain for culture and sensitivity. If the wound becomes infected, the appropriate antibiotic therapy can be instituted.

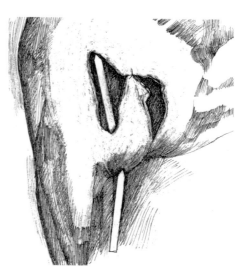

Figure 4-2 Illustration showing the use of a penrose drain in a chest wound.

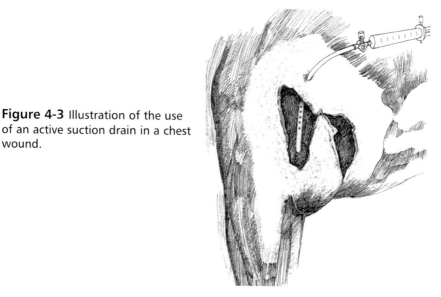

Figure 4-3 Illustration of the use of an active suction drain in a chest wound.

Closure Techniques for Primary Wound Closure

✓ Many options are available for wound closure including suture, staples, and tissue adhesives. The most commonly used technique for wound closure is suturing.

Suture Closure

✓ The choice of suture material is often determined by personal preference. Like many things in life, the choice is not always based upon what is best for the patient, but what is most desired by the practitioner. Suture companies have spent years developing better suture materials that are appropriate for the job at hand. It behooves the practitioner to understand the pros and cons of each suture material before using it then make the best choice based upon the patient.

Needle Type

✓ The type of needle used for suturing is very important in wound closure.

🖉 The practitioner should always strive for the least amount of trauma and inflammation when closing a wound. The reduction in inflammation and trauma will provide a better environment for cosmetic healing.

✓ When suturing skin, a reverse cutting needle is the best choice (Figure 4-4). The needle should be only big enough to allow easy penetration through the skin with minimal tissue drag as the suture is pulled through the needle hole. Sharp needles will always penetrate tissue more easily than dull needles.

✓ Taper-point or taper-cut needles are the most effective for subcutaneous tissue closure.

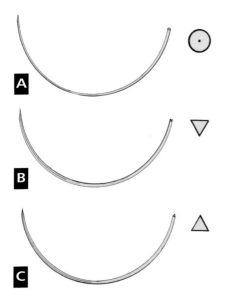

Figure 4-4 Various needles. **A.** Taper point. **B.** Reverse cutting. **C.** Cutting.

✔ One benefit of swaged-on needles is that the needle shaft is contiguous with the suture material. In most cases, the needle diameter is slightly larger than the diameter of the suture material. The result is less trauma to the tissue. These needles will often be sharper than reusable needles since they are only used one time. When using reusable needles, the suture must be passed through the eye of the needle effectively doubling the diameter of material that must be pulled through the tissue. The result is more trauma and consequently inflammation during the healing process (Figure 4-5).

♥ While it may be more expensive to use suture with swaged-on needles than suture from a cassette and reusable needles, in the author's opinion the benefits far outweigh the extra cost. It becomes an issue of doing what is best for the patient, a cost that most of our clients are willing to bear.

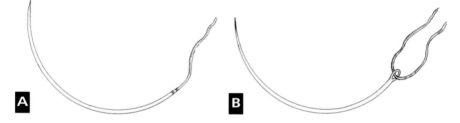

Figure 4-5 A. Swagged-on needle. **B.** Reusable needle. Note doubled diameter of suture on reusable needle.

Absorbable versus Non-absorbable Suture

✔ In general, absorbable sutures should be used when the suture will be buried.

✔ If non-absorbable suture is required for holding strength beyond the typical absorption time, monofilament sutures should be used to minimize the inflammatory response. Monofilament sutures are typically less reactive than braided materials.

✔ Absorbable suture can be used in the skin as long as the client is informed that it may take up to 60 days for the suture to absorb and fall out.

♥ All absorbable suture materials are not created equal. Each tissue in the body will heal within a time frame specific to that tissue. To take advantage of the difference in healing times, suture materials with various absorption times have been developed.

☞ The practitioner should use suture material that will be absorbed from the wound area after the appropriate amount of healing time has elapsed.

♥ The author recommends using synthetic absorbable suture material when the sutures will be buried. In many cases, the faster-absorbing suture materials such as Biosyn (Tyco Healthcare/Kendall) or Monocryl (Ethicon) are very effective in the sub-cutaneous areas (Table 4-1).

Table 4-1
Commonly Used Absorbable and Non-absorbable
Suture Materials

ABSORBABLE (FROM SHORTEST TO LONGEST ABSORPTION TIME)	NON-ABSORBABLE
Monocryl® (Ethicon)	Surgilene® (Tyco Healthcare/Kendall)
Biosyn® (Tyco Healthcare/Kendall)	Monosoft® (Tyco Healthcare/Kendall)
Dexon II® (Tyco Healthcare/Kendall)	Novafil® (Tyco Healthcare/Kendall)
Polysorb® (Tyco Healthcare/Kendall)	Prolene® (Ethicon)
Vicryl® (Ethicon)	Ethibond® (Ethicon)
PDS® (Ethicon)	Ethilon® (Ethicon)
Maxon® (Tyco Healthcare/Kendall)	

Monofilament versus Multifilament Suture

✓ In most cases, monofilament sutures are less reactive and cause less of an inflammatory response than do braided sutures. For this reason, the author uses monofilament suture material for surgery.

✓ However, monofilament suture material tends to have more memory than does multifilament, and the handling characteristics are generally considered poorer than when using a multifilament suture material. Table 4-2 list commonly used mono- and multifilament materials.

✓ Monofilament suture material will often create less tissue drag than will a multifilament suture material.

✋ It has been suggested that multifilament suture material has an increased possibility of wicking bacteria and other contaminants than a monofilament suture material.

☞ When closing skin, a monofilament suture material should be used to reduce the chance of wicking bacteria into the depths of the wound.

✋ This is especially important when suturing skin over a synovial membrane or surgical implant.

Table 4-2.
Commonly Used Monofilament and Multifilament Suture Materials

MONOFILAMENT	MULTIFILAMENT
Biosyn™ (Tyco Healthcare/Kendall)	Polyosorb™ (Tyco Healthcare/Kendall)
Maxon™ (Tyco Healthcare/Kendall)	Dexon II™ (Tyco Healthcare/Kendall)
Surgilene™ (Tyco Healthcare/Kendall)	Vicryl™ (Ethicon)
Monosoft™ (Tyco Healthcare/Kendall)	Ethibond™ (Ethicon)
Novafil™ (Tyco Healthcare/Kendall)	
PDS™ (Ethicon)	
Prolene™ (Ethicon)	
Ethilon™ (Ethicon)	

Suture Patterns for Primary Wound Closure

Appositional Patterns

✓ Appositional patterns are generally considered the gold standard of skin closure. In theory, the tissue layers in the wound are reapposed in the correct anatomical fashion, leading to the most cosmetic and functional end result. The following are types of appositional patterns.

Simple Interrupted Suture Pattern

✓ The simple interrupted suture pattern (Figure 4-6) has often been considered the gold standard of appositional suture patterns. It is an appositional pattern that is easy to place and provides good cosmetic results. Tension along the suture line is limited to each individual suture placed, but if a single suture breaks, the rest of the sutures will generally remain intact.

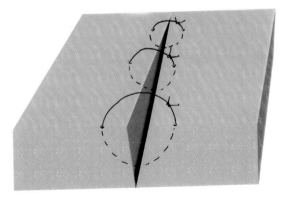

Figure 4-6 A simple interrupted suture pattern.

✂ A simple interrupted pattern should be used in any location where individual sutures may need to be removed to provide better drainage or where the opposing sides of the incision are of unequal length.

✓ The first suture is placed in the center of both sides of the incision or wound. The next two sutures are repeatedly placed in the center of the remaining incision on both sides of the first suture until the wound is closed (Figure 4-7). This will reduce the problem of "dog ears" and leave a more cosmetic result. If necessary, tension-relieving sutures can be placed in the same fashion.

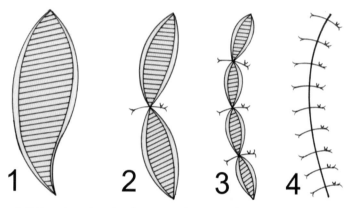

Figure 4-7 Drawing showing how to split an uneven incision in even portions for a cosmetic closure.

✓ A simple interrupted suture line will take longer to place since a knot will have to be tied for each suture. Simple interrupted suture patterns should not be used for buried sutures unless absolutely necessary since the amount of foreign material is dramatically increased in the wound.

✋ Simple interrupted sutures are not good for relieving tension.

Simple Continuous Suture Pattern

✓ The simple continuous suture pattern (Figure 4-8) has many of the same characteristics of the simple interrupted pattern.

✂ The main difference is that the continuous suture is better at equalizing tension across the suture line and it is also faster to place, requiring fewer knots.

✂ If the suture line is to be buried and there is minimal tension on the line, a simple continuous pattern will leave less foreign material in the wound area.

✓ Simple continuous suture lines in the skin are less cosmetic than are interrupted patterns.

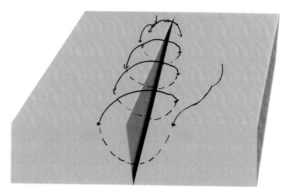

Figure 4-8 A simple continuous suture pattern.

Interlocking Suture Pattern

✓ The interlocking suture pattern (Figure 4-9) offers similar benefits to the simple continuous pattern.

☞ One advantage over a simple continuous pattern is that, in theory, if one loop of suture breaks, the rest of the line will stay intact due to friction of the interlocking loops.

☞ An interlocking suture pattern should not be used if excess tension exists. The locking portion of the pattern runs parallel to the skin edge and, consequently, perpendicular to the vascular supply.

✋ This pattern should be reserved for use in the skin as the amount of foreign material would be unacceptable if buried in a wound.

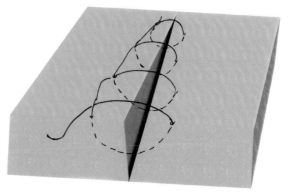

Figure 4-9 An interlocking suture pattern.

Intradermal Suture Pattern

✓ The intradermal suture pattern (Figure 4-10) is a continuous pattern similar to the simple continuous pattern except no suture material is seen at the skin surface.

🔒 It should not be used where there is excess tension. Cosmetic results are generally excellent as long as suture is of the appropriate size.

✓ Large sutures will cause a more severe inflammatory response and a less cosmetic result.

✓ If the suture breaks, the entire line is generally lost.

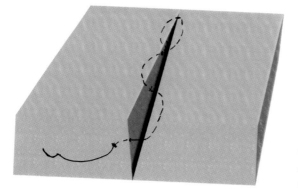

Figure 4-10
An intradermal suture pattern.

Tension-Relieving Suture Patterns

✓ Some suture patterns are better at relieving tension than others. These types of sutures are very important in wounds where there will be more tension on the skin edges. It is common to have some tension in wounds that are closed primarily.

🔒 The amount of tension will often determine not only the type of tension-relieving suture, but the number as well.

🔒 Larger diameter suture material is used to reduce the chance of suture "pull-through".

♥ Use only the amount of tension relieving sutures that are necessary.

✓ In most cases, appositional sutures will be used in conjunction with the tension relieving sutures. Types of tension-relieving sutures follow.

Cruciate Suture Pattern

✓ The cruciate suture pattern (Figure 4-11) is very similar to the simple interrupted pattern. The main difference is that half the number of knots are needed than with the simple interrupted.

✓ There is a minimal increase in tension-relieving ability.

🖐 Cruciate sutures are generally used when there is minimal tension at the skin edges.

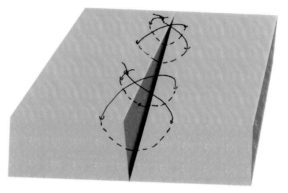

Figure 4-11 A cruciate suture pattern.

Near-Far-Far-Near Suture Pattern

✓ The near-far-far-near suture pattern (Figure 4-12) is an effective tension-relieving pattern. The pattern is easy to apply and never requires the practitioner to pass the needle backwards.

☞ The author prefers this suture pattern because it not only relieves tension, but it also apposes the skin.

✓ The suture runs parallel to the blood supply to the wound edge reducing the likelihood of ischemic necrosis.

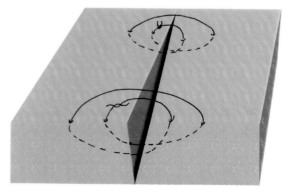

Figure 4-12 A near-far-far-near suture pattern.

Vertical Mattress Suture Pattern

✓ The vertical mattress suture pattern (Figure 4-13) is an effective tension-relieving pattern.

☙ This pattern causes eversion of the skin edge, which will lead to a less cosmetic result. The practitioner is also required to place two suture bites backwards.

✓ The pattern can be used with stents if excess tension is present which reduces the strain on the tissue.

✓ The suture runs parallel to the blood supply to the wound edge, reducing the likelihood of ischemic necrosis.

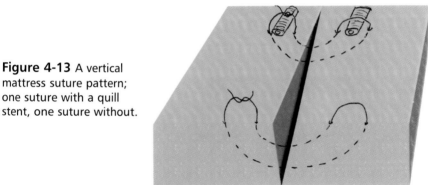

Figure 4-13 A vertical mattress suture pattern; one suture with a quill stent, one suture without.

Horizontal Mattress Suture Pattern

✓ The horizontal mattress suture pattern (Figure 4-14) is an effective suture pattern for relieving tension but the disadvantages generally outweigh the advantages.

☙ The suture causes eversion leading to a poorer cosmetic result.

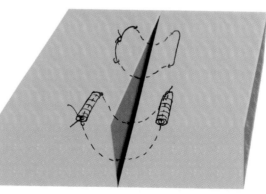

Figure 4-14 A horizontal mattress suture pattern; one suture with a quill stent, one suture without.

🖐 Since part of the suture runs parallel to the skin edge, and consequently, perpendicular to the blood supply, it increases the chance of ischemic necrosis.

✓ The pattern can be used with stents if excess tension is present reducing the strain on the tissue.

Knot Types

🔩 It is important to realize that knot geometry is a very important factor in the volume of suture material that is buried in a wound.

♥ The larger the suture, the greater the volume. The more suture throws, the greater the volume. Using a surgeons throw, the greater the volume (Figure 4-15).

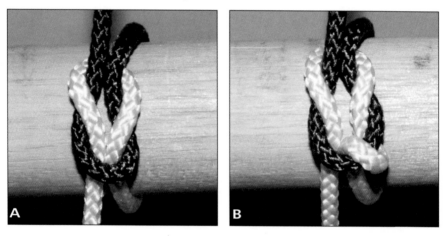

Figure 4-15 The comparison between the geometry of **A.** square knot and **B.** surgeons knot.

🖐 In general, the surgeon should use the smallest size of suture possible with the fewest number of throws and only use a surgeons throw when necessary.

Staple Closure

✓ Stainless steel and titanium staples are available for many different surgical closure options. Staples are very inert and often reduce the surgical time required to close the skin. Skin staples are available in standard and wide widths. Staples do not penetrate the skin very far and consequently provide a reasonable cosmetic result.

✂ Staples can be very effectively used on horses with lacerations at horse shows where local anesthesia is not permitted. The animal can be twitched and the staples applied.

✋ Staples are not recommended in areas where there will be excess tension on the suture line.

✓ Staples are easiest to remove with a staple remover but can be removed with a mosquito forceps (Figure 4-16).

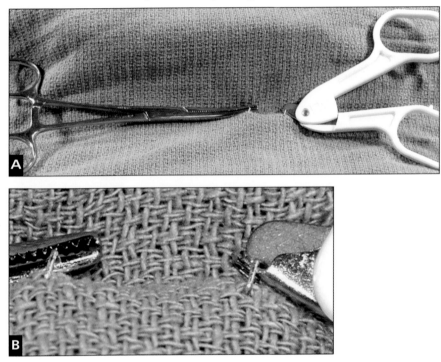

Figure 4-16 A. Staples in a towel showing a staple remover and a Kelly forceps. **B.** Close-up of ends.

Suture/Staple Removal

✓ Sutures and staples are often removed 2 weeks after placement.

✂ This time may be extended if there is tension on the suture line or if the wound is in an area with a lot of movement.

✓ It is rare to leave sutures or staples in for longer than 4 weeks.

✂ In most cases, the tension-relieving sutures can be removed in 2 to 3 weeks and the skin appositional sutures in 3 to 4 weeks.

✋ If sutures are left longer, the greater the risk of an increased inflammatory response and suture sinus infection.

Tissue-Adhesive Closure

✓ Many tissue adhesives are available for wound closure. Most of the adhesives are based upon different formulations of cyanoacrylates. The octylcyanoacrylates are newer formulations that have increased tensile strength with more pliability than the standard cyanoacrylate (Figure 4-17).

🔨 Tissue adhesives can be used on horses with lacerations at horse shows where local anesthesia is not permitted.

✋ Tissue adhesives should not be used in areas where wound tension exists.

✓ The adhesives will break down in 6 to 7 days and should not be used in areas that will have prolonged contact with water.

Figure 4-17
The application of tissue adhesive to a surgical incision.

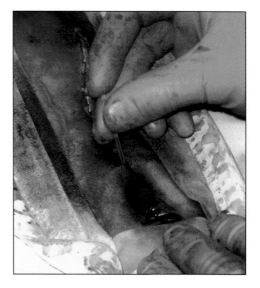

Other Tension-Relieving Techniques

✓ While various tension-relieving sutures can be used to close a wound primarily, it is far more beneficial to actually reduce the amount of tension on the skin.

✓ Undermining of the surrounding skin is the most cosmetic way to reduce tension in a wound (Figure 4-18). In most cases, a combination of blunt and sharp dissection deep to the sub-cutaneous tissue is performed to allow a more tension-free apposition. Care must be taken to leave intact the major arterial supply. If possible, enough undermining should be performed to allow for bringing the skin together without making the surrounding skin look tight.

💣 Excess undermining may lead to skin necrosis.

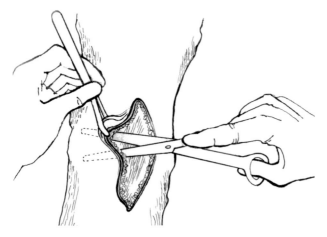

Figure 4-18
Technique to undermine the skin around a wound.

✓ Relief incisions or meshing is another technique for reducing tension in a wound. This should be performed in conjunction with undermining.

☕ The incisions should be made parallel to the original incision. Relief incisions are left to undergo second-intention healing and will therefore often be less cosmetic. In some cases, a single large relief incision is made; in other cases multiple smaller incisions are better (Figure 4-19). In some cases, the relief incisions will allow drainage of dead space as well.

☕ The relief incisions should be made after the wound has been at least partially sutured. This will help the surgeon know how many incisions are necessary.

✋ If the incisions are made incorrectly, disruption of blood supply could be a problem.

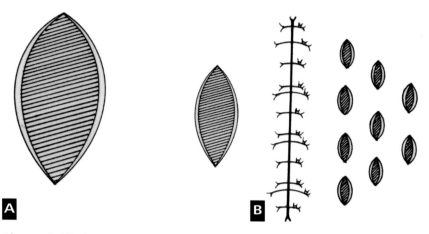

Figure 4-19 The use of relief incisions. **A.** Original wound. **B.** Closed wound with tension-relieving sutures and a single large relief incision on the left side with multiple small relief incisions on the right side.

Wound Protection and Immobilization ⊙

✔ In some areas of the horse, a standard encircling bandage cannot be placed over the wound.

✔ In these areas, a stent can often be used to cover the wound. There are many ways to attach a stent. One way to attach a stent that allows dressing changes is to place individual loop sutures at least 2 inches from the wound edge. These sutures should be placed full thickness through the skin and tied to leave a loop approximately 1 inch in diameter. As many loops as necessary are placed on each side of the wound.

⌘ It is better to err on the side of having too many loops to spread the tension out than too few.

✔ A gauze or towel stent can be placed and held in position using umbilical tape similarly to a shoe lace (Figure 4-20). The stent and underlying dressing can be changed as needed. If there is a lot of exudate, the umbilical tape may need to be replaced during the bandage change. This technique can be used on almost any part of the body.

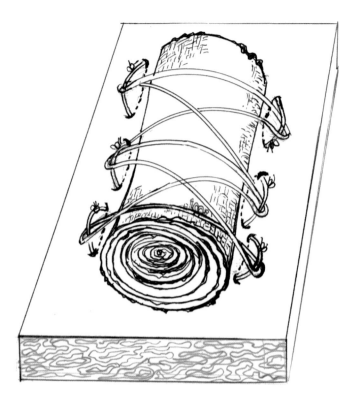

Figure 4-20 A stent applied over a wound.

Specific techniques of wound immobilization are more thoroughly described in Section 1, Wound Care Dressings, Support Dressings.

✓ Wounds that are found over joints or other areas where a lot of motion is possible will often benefit from some type of immobilization. With reduced movement and tension, many wounds will heal more quickly and cosmetically.

✋ It is important to remember that immobilization methods can increase the possibility of pressure sores if not used correctly.

✓ Wounds over the carpus, tarsus, fetlocks, and heels will all heal more rapidly with immobilization (see Figure 4-1).

☞ While cast application may initially be more expensive, it is often more cost effective than placing multiple bandages. As long as the wound can be covered and forgotten for 3 to 4 weeks, a cast is often the most cost effective option.

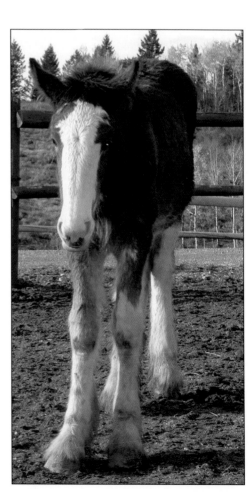

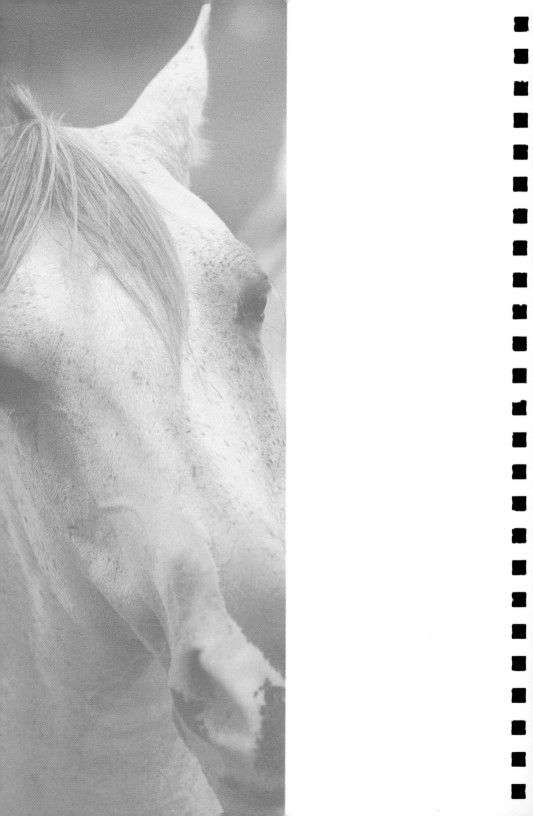

Section 5

Delayed Primary Wound Closure

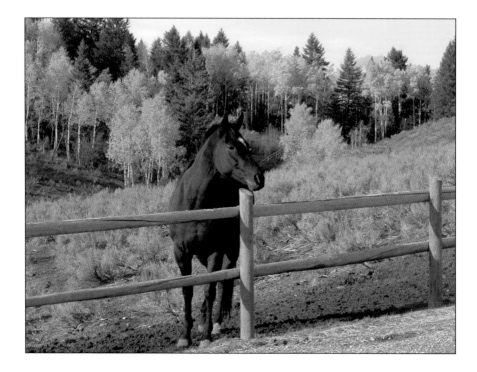

This section will help the practitioner to decide which wounds can be closed in a delayed primary fashion.

Appropriate Wounds

✓ Delayed primary wound closure involves wound closure at any stage where granulation tissue already exists in the wound. This can be accomplished at anytime in the wound healing process, as long as the correct wound environment is present.

☞ There must be enough skin present to allow wound closure with minimal skin tension.

✓ The most common indication for delayed primary closure is a wound where there is too much swelling or contamination to close the wound immediately. With appropriate wound care the swelling and contamination are brought under control and the wound can be closed.

✓ Some wounds become candidates for delayed closure when excess granulation tissue has formed, "ballooning" the skin. When the granulation tissue has been removed, there is often enough skin to allow for primary closure.

♥ The reason for attempting delayed primary closure is to reduce the wound healing time and provide a more cosmetic result for the horse owner. Scaring will generally be kept to a minimum with delayed primary wound closure improving the overall function of the wounded area after healing.

Intermediate Wound Care

✓ Effective wound care should be instituted as soon as possible.

☞ Immediate intervention will generally lead more quickly to a healthy wound bed and, consequently, allow for a more cosmetic and functional closure.

✓ Efforts should be focused on removing devitalized tissue and foreign material, reducing bacterial numbers, and improving the systemic status of the animal as quickly as possible.

☞ Debridement is the most effective method for minimizing foreign material and bacterial numbers.

☞ Antiseptics are generally more traumatic than beneficial to wounds and should be reserved for the peri-wound tissue.

☞ Topical and systemic antibiotics or antimicrobials may speed the reduction in bacterial numbers.

☞ A wound should not be closed until there are less than 10^5 bacteria per gram of tissue. This can be determined with biopsy and quantitative bacteriology, but in most cases a subjective assessment based on the appearance of the wound will be effective.

💣 Skin closure over an infected wound bed will provide an opportunity for an abscess to form, leading to incisional dehiscence.

💣 A thorough examination should be performed to make sure there is no foreign material in the wound, and that vital structures such as tendons or synovial structures have been repaired.

☞ Wound cleansing and debridement are more thoroughly discussed in Section 2, Wound Preparation, Cleaning, and Debridement. The concepts for wound-healing used during this time period are the same as for wounds undergoing second-intention healing. This is discussed in detail in Section 6, Second-Intention Wound Healing.

Preparation for Closure

✓ As soon as the wound bed is healthy, the veterinarian must decide if there is enough skin to close the defect without excess tension.

☞ It is important to remember that in more chronic wounds with excess granulation tissue, the skin may have expanded to cover the extra tissue (Figure 5-1). In these cases, there will be more skin available for closure when the granulation tissue has been removed. If there is enough skin to close without excess tension, it is time to proceed. If there is excess granulation tissue but not enough skin to close without excess tension, the excess granulation tissue should be debulked and moist wound healing techniques continued.

✓ The first step in preparing the wound for closure is to freshen the skin edges. The edges of the skin should be sharply debrided to provide the best opportunity for cosmetic skin healing.

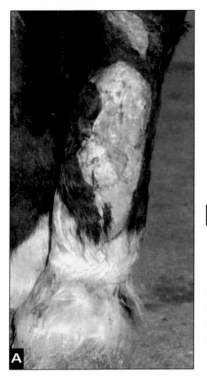

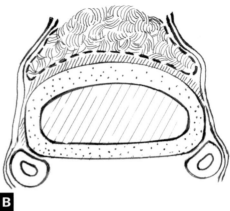

Figure 5-1 A. A chronic wound with granulation tissue ballooning skin. **B.** Drawing of similar wound showing cross section of leg and dashed line to guide removal of granulation tissue.

✓ In many cases the granulation tissue is very vascular. Application of a tourniquet will provide a better field to work in but may obscure the practitioner's ability to determine accurately the junction between normal and abnormal tissue (Figure 5-2).

✓ If the wound is fresh, minimal debridement of the skin edge is generally necessary. If the wound is more chronic, more tissue is removed to facilitate healing. The skin should be undermined to reduce the amount of tension on the wound closure. A combination of sharp and mostly blunt dissection should be performed deep to the sub-cutaneous tissue plane (Figure 5-3).

✋ Undermining too close to the skin or being too aggressive may compromise the blood supply to the skin, leading to ischemic necrosis and incisional dehiscence.

✓ The granulation tissue should be debulked regardless of the amount of tissue present. Often granulation tissue will harbor a large number of bacteria even though there is no clinical indication of bacterial infection. Removing the superficial layers of granulation tissue will remove the superficial bacterial burden, reducing the likelihood of wound infection. The reduction in granulation tissue volume will also reduce the amount of skin

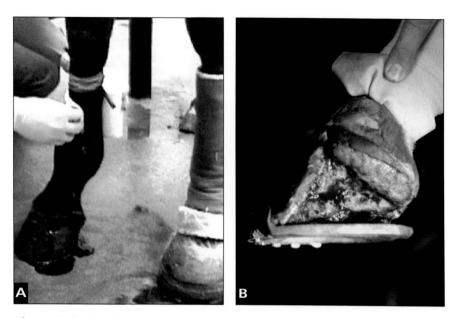

Figure 5-2 Tourniquets. **A.** Surgical tubing on mid cannon, **B.** Eschmarch's bandage on distal cannon and fetlock.

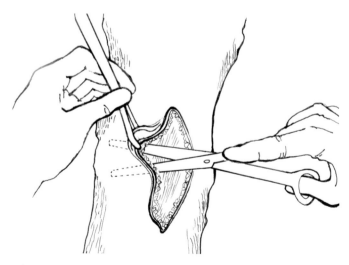

Figure 5-3 Drawing of undermining skin.

necessary to cover the wound and thereby reduce the tension on the skin. A tourniquet will help to provide better visualization and more accurate debridement (Figure 5-4).

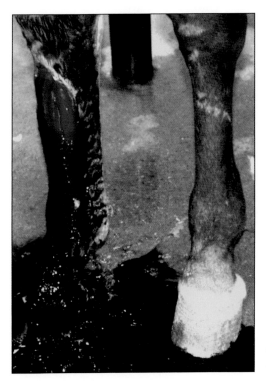

Figure 5-4
Trimming granulation tissue without a tourniquet.

✓ After the granulation tissue has been removed, it is time to close the skin. Further undermining may be performed. If the skin can be apposed with minimal tension, it is time to suture the wound.

✂ If excess tension is still present, other tension-relieving procedures should be used (see Section 4, Primary Wound Closure). In some cases only part of the wound can be closed (Figure 5-5).

✂ As many layers as possible should be closed in order to reduce the amount of dead space and tension on the skin layer.

✓ If necessary either a passive or an active drain should be placed to drain the dead space that can not be closed.

⊙ For information on suture choices, suture patterns, wound protection, and immobilization see Section 4, Primary Wound Closure.

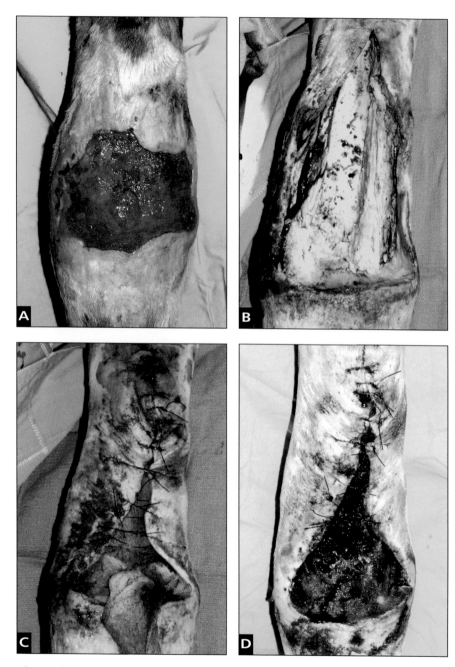

Figure 5-5 A chronic wound where only part of the wound is closed in a delayed primary closure technique. **A.** Wound at presentation, **B.** Wound after granulation tissue has been debulked, **C.** Wound partially closed using tension relieving sutures (near-far-far-near pattern) and packed with moistened antimicrobial roll gauze, **D.** Wound 3 days after surgery at bandage change.

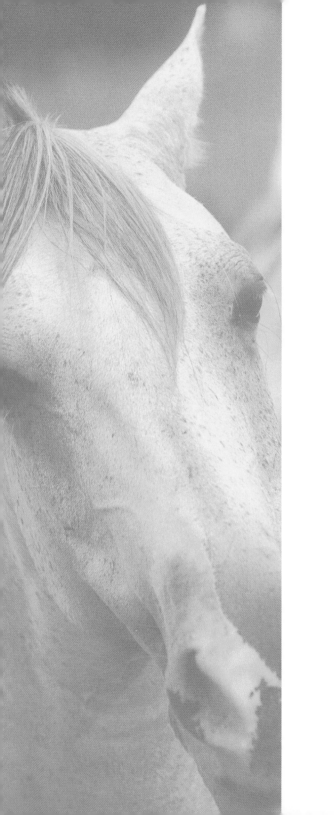

Section 6

Second-Intention Healing

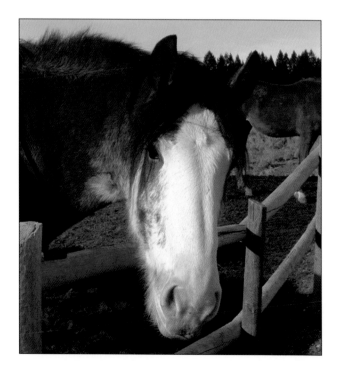

This section will describe the concepts of moist wound healing as they pertain to second-intention healing. The practitioner will be provided with case examples using different wound care products.

✓ Second-intention healing is essentially healing that occurs without surgical attempts to close the wound.

⚷ It is generally reserved for wounds that are grossly contaminated, have large amounts of necrotic debris, or have lost a large enough volume of tissue to make surgical closure impossible.

✓ Second-intention healing will often involve dressings during the course of healing. In the past, the dressing choice has been based more on tradition than scientific evidence. Many different types of dressings have been used including dust, feathers, wool, cotton, oils, salves, ointments, powders, collagen gels, naturally occurring products such as porcine small intestinal sub-mucosa, and, more recently, various synthetic materials. Other topical agents have been used including collagens and growth factors.

✓ In many situations within the equine veterinary field, the standard of care has been to keep the wound clean and dry.

♥ There is now an abundance of evidence indicating that keeping the wound moist will provide the best environment for optimal wound healing, and will provide faster and more cosmetic wound healing.

Moist-Wound Healing Concepts

♥ Moist-wound healing is a relatively new concept in medicine and occurs when the wound exudate is allowed to stay in contact with the wound bed. While this has certainly occurred in veterinary medicine, it is often more by accident than design. Dressings are left on longer than planned because of the inconvenience of getting them changed and the wound exudate has the opportunity to stay next to the wound bed.

✓ George Winter is often credited with beginning the moist-wound healing revolution. Winter in 1962 showed that full-thickness skin wounds in both swine and humans kept in a moist environment re-epithelialize in approximately 12 to 15 days, while the same wound exposed to the air took 25-30 days to heal. The wounds were less inflamed, caused less itching, had less eschar formation, and were more likely to heal without scarring.

✓ While Winter often gets the credit, work by Bloom and Bull preceded his report. Bloom was an army surgeon who sterilized cellophane and used it as a semipermeable membrane to treat burn wounds at a World War II prisoner of war camp. His primary goal was to reduce the risk of bacteria entering the wound. He found his patients were able to move without the pain that patients with other dressings had. There was less loss of plasma from the patient, and infection seemed to be reduced. The dressings were very effective, but being made of rubber they were occlusive, retaining too much fluid. The surrounding skin would often become macerated. Bull in 1948, began studying a transparent nylon dressing. The dressing stopped bacterial and fluid penetration, but did not allow fluid collection and maceration of the normal skin. In a large study using the transparent nylon dressing with an adhesive, wounds healed faster and required fewer dressing changes.

☞ The principles of moist-wound healing suggest that wound exudate will provide the necessary cells, and a substrate rich in enzymes, growth factors, and chemotactic factors that will control infection and provide the best environment for healing. The enzymes are a byproduct of both the breakdown of polymorphonuclear cells and macrophages, and from tissue release in the form of metalloproteinases. Occlusion maintains contact of the enzymes and metalloproteinases to the wound surface, leading to debridement of devitalized tissue, improving the "foundation" for wound healing to proceed. This has been termed "autolytic debridement." Autolytic debridement begins between 72 and 96 hours after beginning treatment of a dry wound, depending upon the thickness of eschar and the size/location of the wound, and is achieved under occlusive dressings provided the wound fluid remains in contact with the wound bed.

✋ It is therefore important not to let the wound bed become dry, or it will slow the healing process.

☞ Growth factors and cytokines provide a stimulus for the fibroblasts, epithelial cells, and angiogenesis. The chemotactic factors stimulate the migration of more neutrophils and macrophages to phagocytize bacteria and debris, while releasing enzymes to further promote autolytic debridement. A moist environment allows better migration of neutrophils and macrophages than a dry wound environment. Occlusion provides a constant thermally regulated environment, leading to healthier cells. If the appropriate dressing is chosen, bacterial penetration is reduced or prevented.

♥ Disadvantages of moist healing include bacterial colonization, folliculitis, the possibility of trauma to peri-ulcer borders, and, at least in people, allergies to the dressing material.

♥ It is important to realize that if the wound tissue is not infected prior to occlusion, it is unlikely that it will become so using an occlusive dressing. It is quite probable that a moist environment with increased cellular components will actually reduce the number of micro-organisms present in a wound. In one study, it was determined that wound fluid has bacteriostatic to mildly bactericidal activity. It is possible that the wound fluid will also act as a bacterial barrier. Frequent dressing changes provide access of more airborne bacteria to the wound surface. Moist-wound healing techniques often reduce the frequency of dressing changes, thereby reducing the chance of airborne bacteria contamination or infection.

💣 There is a fine balance between drying out the wound and maceration of peri-wound tissue. This balance will change often during the stages of wound healing. Moist wounds are still considered to be less painful than dry wounds, especially during dressing changes.

✋ While the concept of moist-wound healing may seem somewhat daunting, there are new dressings available to help the practitioner in determining what to use in each case to provide an optimum wound-healing environment (Table 6-1).

Table 6-1
Advantages and Disadvantages of Moist Wound Healing

ADVANTAGES	DISADVANTAGES
Rapid autolytic debridement	Bacterial colonization
Less necrotic tissue	Folliculitis
Bacterial barrier	Possible trauma to peri-ulcer borders
Waterproof barrier	Allergies to the dressing material (in people)
Decrease in pain associated with wound/dressing	
Ease of use	
Fewer dressing changes	
Decreased wound-healing time	

♥ To appropriately use wound care dressings the practitioner must understand that the wound will have different characteristics during different healing stages. The characteristics of the wound immediately after the traumatic incident will vary depending upon the type of trauma associated. With sharp trauma the wound will generally have less necrotic tissue than with blunt trauma. Regardless, the wound will start out moist. Wounds with an excess of necrotic tissue will generally have more exudate than wounds with minimal necrotic tissue. As the wound progresses, it is either kept moist or allowed to dry out. Moist wounds will eventually move from the clean-up stage to the granulating and contraction stage. Eventually wounds will epithelialize.

Each of the different stages will be best addressed by a specific dressing type.

Dressing Choices

✓ Many dressings have been used in the treatment of lacerations and abrasions in horses.

☞ It is important to remember that a dressing might take the form of anything from gauze to ointments, and injections of plasma rich-protein.

✓ Non-adherent dressings and gauze dressings are probably the most commonly used dressings. Both of these dressings are porous, allowing fluid transfer from the wound to the overdressing, and from the outside of the bandage to the wound surface (Figure 6-1).

☞ With woven gauze, the wound exudate is quickly absorbed through the gauze and into the over dressing. This is termed "vertical wicking".

☞ If non-woven gauze is used, the wound exudate tends to flow to the edge of the gauze quickly and then is absorbed into the over dressing. This is termed "horizontal wicking".

♥ The amount of moisture retention is dependent upon many factors, including the amount of exudate and the type of gauze, the secondary dressing, and the frequency of dressing change.

It is difficult when using a gauze dressing to maintain a moist wound-healing environment, even if a "wet to dry" dressing is used. In many cases, the gauze will need to be remoistened frequently, as often as 4 to 6 times per day, to maintain moisture.

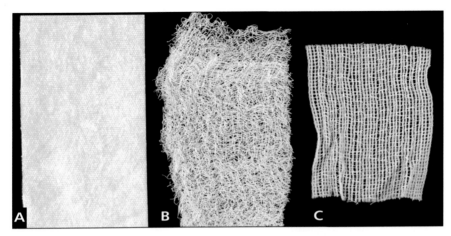

Figure 6-1 Primary dressings. **A.** Non-adherent dressing (Telfa™ Tyco Healthcare/Kendall). **B.** Woven gauze. **C.** Non-woven gauze.

✓ Non-adherent dressings such as the Telfa™ pad (Tyco Healthcare/Kendall) have long been considered the gold standard in equine wound care (see Figure 6-1). They are easy to apply and are readily available, making them a common choice in veterinary care. While in the past they have played a role in wound healing, new dressings that have been manufactured for specific wound-healing stages will generally provide better results.

♥ The concept of using a single dressing throughout the entire wound-healing process is outdated. The practitioner must understand that the wound changes frequently and that the wound requirements can be best met by using different wound-care products throughout the healing process.

✓ Occlusive dressings isolate the wound from the external environment, providing many benefits over gauze dressings (Figure 6-2). The occlusiveness of a dressing is measured by the evaporation of fluids from the wound surface through the dressing, and ranges from minimally occlusive to completely occlusive.

☞ The benefits of occlusion include rapid autolytic debridement with less necrotic tissue, a bacterial barrier, a waterproof barrier, a decrease in pain associated with wound/dressing, ease of use, fewer dressing changes, and decreased wound-healing time.

✓ Many practitioners fear the development of infection when using occlusive dressings. All wounds are colonized with bacteria but they may not actually be infected. In general infection refers

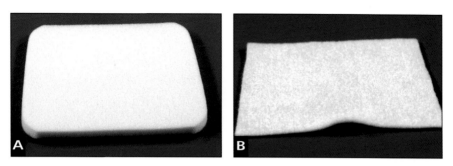

Figure 6-2 Occlusive dressings. **A.** Semi-occlusive foam dressing (Hydrasorb™ Tyco Healthcare/Kendall). **B.** Calcium alginate dressing.

to invasion of 10^5 bacteria per gram of tissue. Signs of infection include edema, erythema, induration, and fever. While there are concerns, studies have shown that occlusive dressings are not associated with increased rates of infection.

The ideal dressing should keep the wound bed continually moist and the surrounding skin dry, or, more simply, manage the amount of exudate present. This determination depends on good clinical judgment.

♥ It is important to understand that the future in equine wound care is most likely in the use of multiple dressings used throughout the healing process. Most dressings address specific needs and have been designed to achieve specific results. Gone are the days when a single dressing type is used throughout the entire wound-healing process.

✓ The dressings described in this section are hypertonic saline dressings, antimicrobial dressings, hydragels, calcium alginate dressings, collagen and maltodextran dressings, various replacement dressings, growth factors, semi-occlusive foam dressings, and steroids. These dressings are discussed in the sequential order a practitioner might use them during the wound-healing process.

Hypertonic Saline Dressing ⊙

✓ Hypertonic saline dressings (Figure 6-3) have been designed for use on necrotic or heavily exuding wounds. The hypertonic saline works by osmotic action to desiccate the necrotic tissue and bacteria in a wound.

The debridement is non-selective and must be carefully monitored to ensure the surrounding tissue is not damaged.

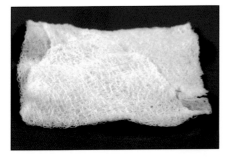

Figure 6-3 Hypertonic saline dressing.

✔ Dressings should be changed every 24 to 48 hours at the onset on treatment. The hypertonicity and, consequently, the efficacy of the dressing will be reduced in the face of heavy exudate. As the exudate decreases, the frequency of dressing can be reduced. This type of dressing has been effectively used in chronic abscesses such as those caused by Corynebacterium pseudotuberculosis (Figure 6-4). The author prefers to use Curasalt™ (Tyco Healthcare/Kendall), a loosely woven gauze dressing premoistened with 20% hypertonic saline. This dressing has been more effective in removing necrotic tissue and reducing the bacterial load than gauze moistened with 7.5% or 10% hypertonic saline.

☞ Once the necrotic tissue has been removed and bacterial infection is no longer an issue, another dressing type such as a calcium alginate or semi-occlusive foam dressing should be used.

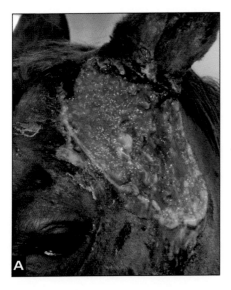

Figure 6-4
A horse with *Corynebacterium* pseudo-tuberculosis infection near left ear. **A.** 24 hours after presentation having just removed a non-adherent dressing. **B.** Wound after 2 days of hypertonic saline dressing therapy. **C.** Wound after a total of 6 days hypertonic saline dressing therapy and just prior to applying a calcium alginate dressing.

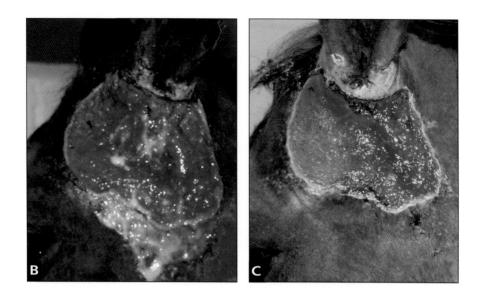

Case Example ♥

Signalment and History: A 6-month-old Appaloosa filly with laceration of the plantar aspect of the mid metatarsus on the left hind leg of 1-month duration. The wound had been treated with standard wound care consisting of a non-adherent dressing and a pressure bandage. Twenty-four hours prior to presentation, the filly had become acutely lame on the leg, and was noted to have fluctuant swellings on the medial and lateral aspects of the leg just dorsal to the previous laceration.

Clinical Examination: On clinical examination of the leg, there were necrotic areas involving the skin and subcutaneous tissues just dorsal to the original laceration. These areas of necrotic, hemorrhagic tissue were considered secondary to a dissecting septic cellulitis, presumably associated with an infection of the original wound and subsequent granulation tissue. The granulation tissue associated with the original laceration was noted to be edematous and exuberant. The distal cannon region was swollen, and the foal would only occasionally bear weight.

Presentation: The wounds were cleaned with dilute betadine scrub using woven gauze for debridement and the area was rinsed with sterile saline (Figure 6-5). A Curasalt™ (hypertonic saline) dressing was applied to the leg, covering all of the affected areas to provide autolytic debridement and assist in the removal of the necrotic tissue. The Curasalt™ dressing was held intact with Kerlix A.M.D.™ roll gauze (antimicrobial dressing used to provide a barrier to bacterial penetration) which was subsequently moistened with sterile saline. To maintain a moist environment, the dressings were covered with a rectal sleeve. A standard pressure bandage was placed over the wound dressing and left in place for 24 hours. The foal was not started on systemic antibiotics or anti-inflammatory medications.

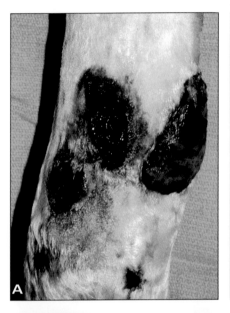
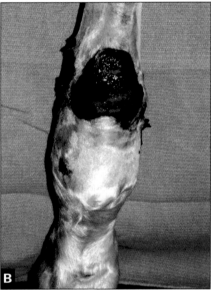
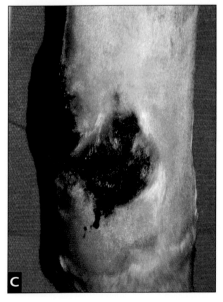

Figure 6-5 The paint foal at presentation. **A.** Lateral view. **B.** Plantar view. **C.** Medial view.

24 hours: The wound was rinsed with sterile saline, and the area was once again debrided with woven gauze (Figure 6-6) with dressings applied in a similar manner. At this time, the swelling in the leg had reduced, and the foal was beginning to use the leg.

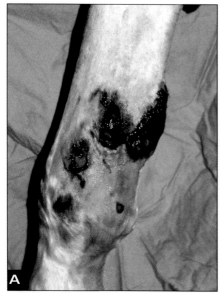

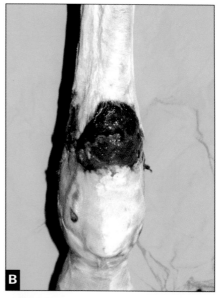

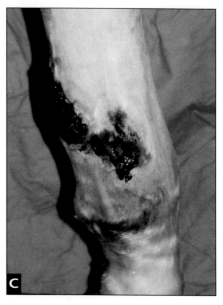

Figure 6-6 The paint foal at 24 hours after hypertonic saline dressing therapy. **A.** Lateral view. **B.** Plantar view. **C.** Medial view.

96 hours: The bandage and dressings were removed and the wound rinsed with sterile saline (Figure 6-7). The abscess sites and the original wound were filled with healthy pink granulation tissue.

There was no evidence of bacterial infection, and the amount of exudate was minimal. At this point, the medial and lateral wounds were covered with moistened calcium alginate dressings (Curasorb™) to stimulate further granulation tissue, and the original plantar wound was covered with Hydrasorb to reduce the exuberant granulation tissue. The swelling in the leg had completely resolved, and the foal would bear weight normally.

Table 6-2 shows which wound types respond to hypertonic saline.

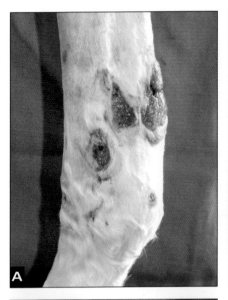

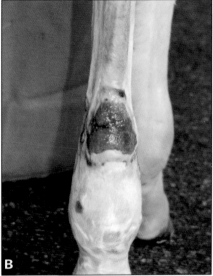

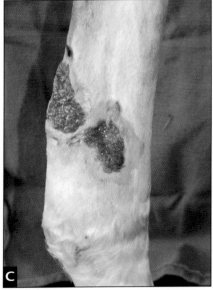

Figure 6-7 The paint foal at 96 hours after hypertonic saline dressing therapy. **A.** Lateral view. **B.** Plantar view. **C.** Medial view.

Table 6-2
Wound Types for Hypertonic Saline Dressings

Heavily exudative wounds

Necrotic wounds

Infected wounds

Anti-Microbial Dressings ⊙

✓ A new concept in wound care is the anti-microbial dressing, where a dressing material is impregnated with an anti-microbial agent.

☙ These agents are not antiseptics and, consequently, cause less trauma to the wound-healing cells than antiseptics.

✓ Gauze dressings like Kerlix A.M.D.™ (Tyco Healthcare/Kendall) are bound with an anti-microbial agent and have been designed to provide a barrier to bacterial penetration and, hence, colonization. Kerlix A.M.D.™ contains polyhexamethylene biguanide (PHMB) bound to a Kerlix Super Sponge™. PHMB is part of a class of cationic surface-active agents that have been used as preservatives in aqueous solutions and as disinfectants and antiseptics. Current uses of PHMB include cosmetics, contact lens solutions, baby wipes, and pool sanitizers. Increased concentrations, when impregnated into fabric, have shown the ability to suppress microbial growth and penetration. Microbial death occurs by destabilization and disruption of the cytoplasmic membrane, resulting in leakage of macromolecular components. This response is irreversible, and the microbe cannot adapt or become "resistant" to the PHMB. These dressings are particularly useful in preventing bacterial infection in surgical incisions or where wounds are close to synovial structures and subsequent deep penetration of bacteria would be catastrophic (Figure 6-8). The Kerlix A.M.D.™ is packaged in both a Super Sponge gauze as well as Roll Gauze.

✓ Studies were performed on swine after creating full-thickness wounds on each side of the body, covering the wounds with plain gauze and gauze impregnated with an antimicrobial respectively. Bacteria were then placed over the gauze and the wound site cultured. The antimicrobial gauze stopped all bacterial penetration, while the plain gauze did not stop any bacterial penetration.

☙ When used in open wounds, the antimicrobial dressings should be moistened with saline to prevent drying in the wound. The dressings can be used dry over surgically closed wounds.

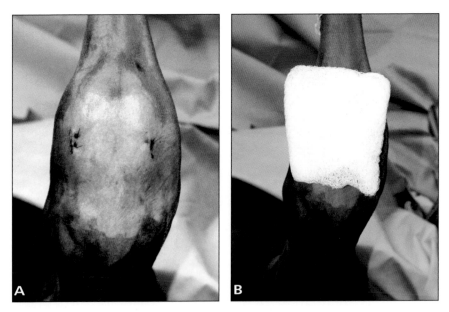

Figure 6-8 A carpus after carpal arthroscopy. **A.** Surgical incisions. **B.** Surgical incisions covered by AMD.

In the author's experience, these dressings will also reduce the bacterial load at the wound site.

Case Example ♥

Signalment and History: A 4-year-old intact female Thoroughbred horse was presented with a 6-month history of having reared up and fallen over backwards.

Clinical Exam: The horse had disfigurement and persistent drainage at the withers (Figure 6-9). Radiographs showed several fractures of the dorsal spinous processes of the withers with signs of sequestration and infection (Figure 6-10).

Treatment: The horse was taken to surgery, and the affected dorsal spinous processes were removed. Three of the spinous processes were obviously sequestered and removed. Two other processes were infected and removed. The wound was lavaged and sharply debrided (Figure 6-11). Kerlix A.M.D. roll gauze was moistened with isotonic saline and placed into the wound to fill dead space (Figure 6-12). Approximately 75% of the wound was closed primarily, leaving a portion of the gauze exiting the wound. A stent was secured over the wound, and the horse recovered from anesthesia (Figure 6-13). The gauze was removed

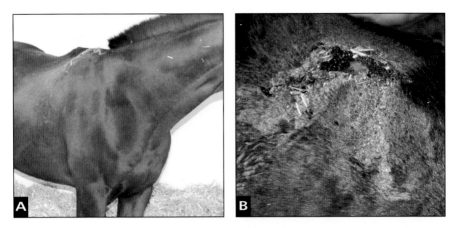

Figure 6-9 A. Horse with septic dorsal spinous process fractures. **B.** Close-up of withers region.

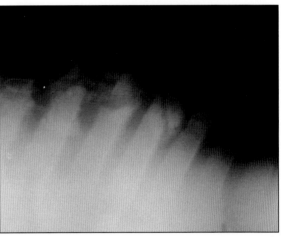

Figure 6-10
Radiograph of the horse in Figure 6-9.

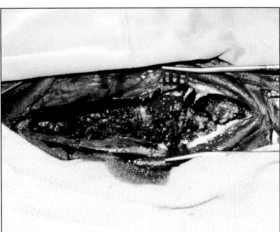

Figure 6-11
Intra-operative picture after fracture removal and wound debridement.

and replaced at 48 hours. There was no sign of infection at the time of dressing change, and the surrounding tissue was consistent with normal healthy granulation tissue. Packing was continued for an additional 72 hours.

✔ Silver has been recently impregnated into dressings and can be used in a similar fashion. The silver impregnated dressings are more expensive.

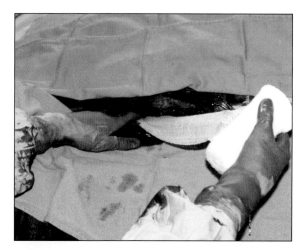

Figure 6-12
Filling of the defect with saline moistened antimicrobial roll gauze.

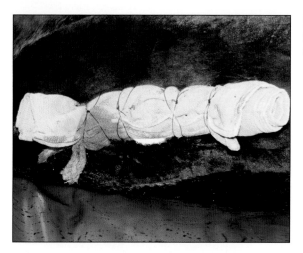

Figure 6-13
Stent placement over the surgically debrided wound.

⚷ The dressings should be changed every 3 to 7 days depending on the amount of exudate.

⚷ Once the wound is clean or the incision has sealed, another dressing type should be used. If there is a deficit of granulation tissue, a calcium alginate dressing is chosen; if the granulation tissue is at the skin surface, a semi-occlusive foam dressing is chosen.

Table 6-3 shows wound types responding to anti-microbial dressings.

Table 6-3
Wound Types for Anti-microbial Dressings

Surgical Incisions
Mild to heavily exudative wounds
Necrotic wounds
Infected wounds
Wounds over a synovial structure

Hydragel Dressings ⊙

✓ Hydragels are moist medical grade gels that create a moist wound-healing environment when used on a dry wound. They are composed of water, glycerin, and a polymer. They are conformable, nondrying, convenient, and bacterial free, and they provide water to the wound surface maintaining a moist environment.

☞ When a wound has a scab, hydragels will promote wound debridement by moistening the scab.

✓ They are available in either an amorphous gel, gel-impregnated gauze, or in a mesh-reinforced pad (Figure 6-14). The gels are completely occlusive and will allow a dry wound to become moist, improving autolytic debridement, white blood cell migration, thermal regulation, and subsequent improved wound healing.

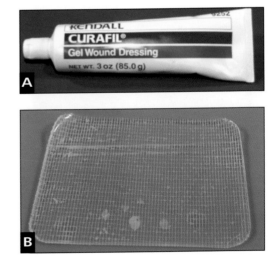

Figure 6-14
A. Amorphous gel (Curafil™, Tyco Healthcare/Kendall).
B. Mesh reinforced gel pad (Curagel™, Tyco Healthcare/Kendall).

🔑 The author uses a hydragel dressing mainly in dry wounds, but they have been used in wounds throughout all stages of healing. They are very useful in painful wounds.

🔑 The dressing should be changed every 4 to 7 days depending on the amount of exudate.

🔑 Once the wound has become moist, the gels are discontinued in favor of one of the other semi-occlusive dressings.

Case Example ♥

Signalment and History: A 5-year-old paint presented with a right hind limb dorsal cannon bone laceration of approximate 2-weeks duration.

Clinical Examination: The horse was in good physical condition with the only abnormality limited to the right hind limb. There was a full thickness degloving type injury to the leg from the distal tarsus to the proximal fetlock. The wound was dry with minimal necrotic tissue at the edges (Figure 6-15).

Treatment: The horse was sedated and the wound filled with KY Jelly. The hair was clipped and the leg explored for any other abnormalities. After thorough examination, the wound was covered

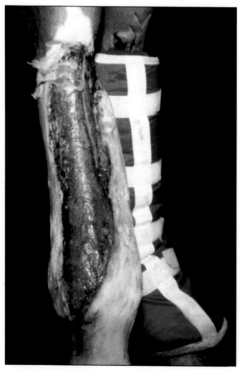

Figure 6-15
A horse with dry right hind cannon laceration with a dry wound bed.

with three hydragel pads. The gel pads were secured with roll gauze and covered with a compression bandage. The dressings were changed in 7 days. At this time, the wound was moist, and autolytic debridement had removed the majority of necrotic debris. Another gel dressing was applied for 7 days. As soon as the wound had moist healthy granulation tissue the dressing type was changed to a calcium alginate dressing.

Wound types for hydragels are shown in Table 6-4.

Table 6-4
Wound Types for Hydragels

Dry wounds
Dry wounds with cavities (amorphous gel)
Minor burns
Abrasions
Minor irritations of the skin
Painful wounds

Calcium Alginate Dressings ⊙

✓ Calcium alginate dressings are soft, non-woven fabric pads composed of sodium and calcium alginate, a derivative of seaweed.

⚡ The calcium in the dressing interacts with sodium in the wound, providing a wound exudate that stimulates the myofibroblasts and the epithelial cells while speeding wound homeostasis. Calcium also serves as a modulator in epithelial cell proliferation and migration.

⚡ The alginate dressing is used in moderately to heavily draining wounds and can absorb up to 20 times its weight in exudate, reducing the frequency of bandage changes.

⚡ The dressing conforms to wound contours, applies easily, and removes virtually painlessly and intact.

⚡ The good vertical wicking properties allow a reduction in maceration of healthy peri-wound tissue.

✓ The alginate dressings come in pads or rope that can be used for loose packing to fill deep wounds (Figure 6-16). They can be trimmed to size and are very conformable. Newer alginate dressings (Curasorb Zn™, Tyco Healthcare/Kendall) are provided with zinc embedded in the dressing which provides necessary elements for epithelialization.

✓ Alginate dressings have been associated with a reduction of pain during dressing changes.

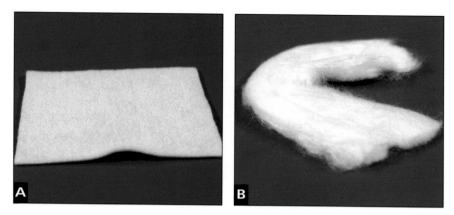

Figure 6-16 Calcium alginate in **A.** pad and **B.** rope.

⚷ In general, the alginates are used after the wound has been debrided and cleaned, or moistened by a gel. Use of alginates will stimulate granulation tissue and prepare the wound bed for a foam dressing.

✋ In wounds that lack excess exudate but still need granulation tissue stimulation, the alginates can be pre-moistened with normal saline prior to application.

⚷ The dressings can be changed every 3 to 7 days depending on the amount of exudate.

Case Example: Dry Wound ♥

Signalment and History: A 5-day-old paint foal was presented for flexural limb deformities of both fore limbs.

Clinical Examination: On presentation, the foal was noted to have full-thickness skin abrasions over the dorsal aspect of both forelimb fetlocks. The affected skin was thickened and devitalized. Kerlix A.M.D.™ Super Sponge was moistened and applied to the affected area to prevent bacterial colonization and subsequent infectious arthritis (Figure 6-17).

Treatment: The wound was covered with Curasorb™, a calcium alginate dressing, and held in place with roll gauze (Figure 6-18). In retrospect, the wound should have been treated with hypertonic saline to remove the eschar prior to calcium alginate application. Because there was minimal exudate, the dressing was moistened with saline (Figure 6-19). If the dressing is not pre-moistened in such cases, the wound bed will become too dry.

Figure 6-17
A distal cannon wound in a young foal prior to alginate application. The wound had been covered with Kerlix A.M.D. for 5 days before this picture was taken.

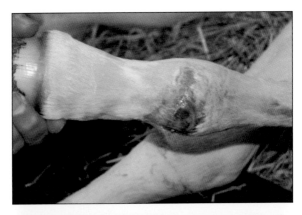

Figure 6-18
Calcium alginate dressing on wound.

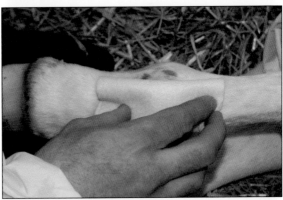

Figure 6-19
Moistening gauze and calcium alginate dressing with saline.

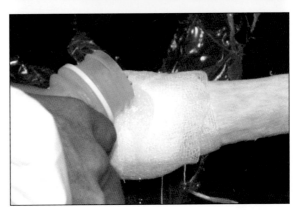

The moistened dressing was covered with plastic to maintain moisture and the plastic was secured with an elastic bandage to minimize slippage (Figure 6-20). The leg was then wrapped with combine cotton, gauze, vet-wrap, and elastacon (Figure 6-21). The dressing was left in place for 5 to 7 days at a time. After three weeks of calcium alginate dressings, the wound was covered with a semi-occlusive foam dressing. The foam dressing was changed every 7 days until the wound healed. This picture was taken 10 weeks after initiation of therapy with Curasorb (Figure 6-22).

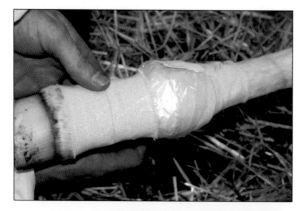

Figure 6-20 Covering a wound with plastic to maintain moisture.

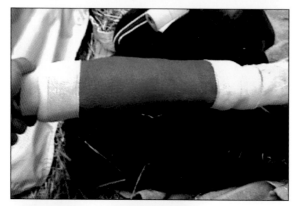

Figure 6-21
The finished bandage.

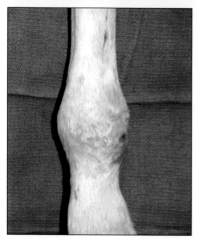

Figure 6-22
The healed wound at 10 weeks after injury.

Case Example: Moist Wound ♥

Signalment and History: An adult horse was presented for a laceration of the right antebrachium.

Clinical Examination: On presentation, the horse was noted to have a non-acute granulating laceration of the right antebrachium. There was a moderate amount of wound exudate and granulation tissue already present. There had been sutures applied to keep a stent bandage in place (Figure 6-23). The wound was cleaned with a surfactant-based wound cleanser (Constant Clens™, Tyco Healthcare/Kendall), and no other mechanical debridement was performed (Figure 6-24).

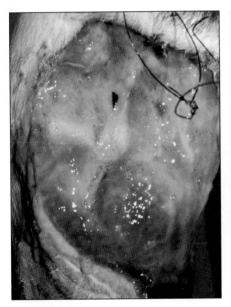 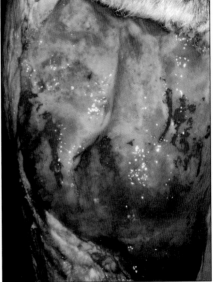

Figure 6-23
Distal-lateral antebrachial wound after bandage removal.

Figure 6-24
Picture of wound after using a surfactant-based wound cleanser (Constant-Clens™ Tyco Healthcare/Kendall).

Treatment: A calcium alginate dressing was placed in the cleft between the two muscle bellies to stimulate better healing and another sheet of calcium alginate dressing was placed directly over the wound to stimulate granulation tissue formation (Table 6-5). There was enough exudate in the wound to negate the need for moistening the alginate dressing (Figure 6-25). The alginate dressing was held in place with Kerlix A.M.D.™ roll gauze (Tyco Healthcare/Kendall) to minimize bacterial penetration.

121

A fairly standard pressure bandage was used over the alginate and antimicrobial dressing. The owner changed the dressing every 4 to 7 days, depending on the amount of exudate present. After the wound had granulated sufficiently, a semi-occlusive foam dressing was used to encourage epithelialization.

Table 6-5
Wound Types for Alginate Dressings

Wounds with moderate to heavy exudate
Dehisced surgical wounds
Abrasions
Pressure ulcers
Wounds where granulation tissue in needed
Wounds with exposed bone

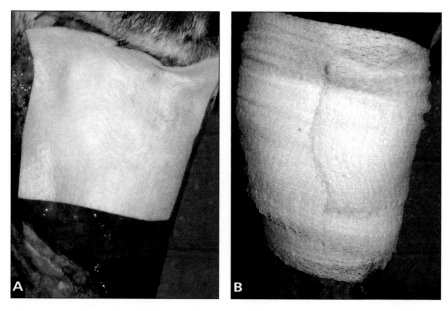

Figure 6-25 Wound dressings. **A.** Calcium alginate dressing. **B.** Antimicrobial roll gauze.

Topical Dressings: Collagens, Maltrodextrans

✓ Collagen is obviously a very important component of normal skin, and consequently, wound healing. The final product in wound healing is dependent on the production, maturation, and degradation of collagen.

✓ The final wound strength will be determined by the character and quality of collagen produced by fibroblasts.

⚡ Exogenous collagen is very hydrophilic, maintaining a moist wound environment and potentially providing a cleaner wound environment. In one study with dogs, the wounds had less inflammation and a greater percentage of epithelialization with collagen treatment.

✓ There are many forms of collagen available including powders, gels, and sponges (Figure 6-26). The benefits of collagen dressings have been attributed to the provision of a scaffold for fibroblasts and a chemotactic agent for white blood cells.

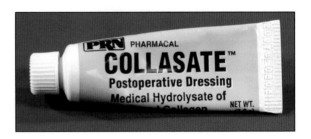

Figure 6-26 A collagen dressing (Collasate™ PRN Pharmacal).

⚡ Collagen dressings are best reserved for the granulation stage of wound healing.

⚡ After adequate granulation tissue has formed, a semi-occlusive foam dressing should be used.

✓ Maltrodextrans are polysaccharide powders obtained from plant starches. In in vitro studies, they have been shown to inhibit the growth of some bacteria, including *Psuedomonas aeruginosa, Staphlococcus aureus* and *Bacteroides fragilis*. While the exact mechanism is unclear it seems to be due to an alteration in cell wall function.

✓ It has been proposed that maltrodextrans will provide nutrition to the wound healing cells in the form of glucose. In a pilot study in horses, maltrodextran provided better tissue healing results than did nitrofurazone. Dressings are available as powders and gels (Figure 6-27).

⚡ These dressings are probably best reserved for the granulating stage of wound healing (Table 6-6).

⚡ Once adequate granulation tissue is present, a semi-occlusive foam dressing should be used.

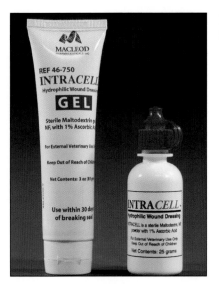

Figure 6-27 Maltrodextran dressings (Intracell MacLeod Pharmaceuticals).

Table 6-6
Wound Types for Collagen and Maltrodextran Dressings

Wounds in the granulation stage of healing after infection and necrotic debris in the wound have been reduced.

Replacement Tissue Dressings

✓ Various substances have been used recently as replacement type dressings.

☞ These dressings have been designed to provide a framework over which other cells migrate and as a stimulant to those cells to form the tissue that is desired.

✓ While these have only begun to be used in the equine arena, it is important to recognize that they are available.

☞ Porcine small intestinal submucosa has been used primarily to replace lost vessels and to repair intestinal defects. Recently clinical studies in small animals have shown promise in treating bone defects in the skull, tendon injury, and skin wounds. It is critical to keep the tissue replacement moist.

☞ ACell (ACell, Inc) is a naturally occurring extracellular matrix scaffold from the bladder that was designed to promote the repair and replacement of tissue much like porcine small intestinal submucosa. The concept associated with ACell is that the tissue replacement provides structural and functional proteins that influence how cells attach, express their genes, and eventually differentiate. In experimental studies, the material has been shown to affect the type of cells recruited. Studies have also shown that the tissue is not rejected by the host unlike other xenographic transplants, and that they are eventually completely replaced by host cells. Tissue types that have invaded the membrane experimentally include: urinary tract, dura mater, esophagus, musculotendinous tissues, and blood vessels. One study has shown an antimicrobial activity to the biomaterials. ACell has been used in a number of clinical wound cases with positive results. The end result of the wound is often very normal in character and function. Both substances are completely replaced by the host's normal tissue (Table 6-7).

Table 6-7
Wound Types for Tissue Replacement/Scaffold Dressings

Wounds with tissue defects.
Wounds undergoing granulation.

✔ While little research has been done in the horse, it would benefit the practitioner to keep apprised of these types of dressings in the future.

✔ The use of equine amnion has been used sporadically on equine wounds. Amnion is considered a biological dressing similar to ACell and porcine small intestinal submucosa.

🔑 Studies have shown that the use of equine amnion reduces wound retraction and granulation tissue formation and improves epithelialization. It has also been shown beneficial for use in skin grafting as a non-adherent dressing.

🔑 The main drawback to amnion is the availability and the amount of time necessary for preparation.

Growth Factors

✔ Growth factors have become very popular in experimental studies for repairing wound tissue.

🔑 Cytokines have been shown to have chemotactic effects, mitogenic effects, and activating effects which simulate production of the extracellular matrix components. Studies have shown the benefit of platelet-derived growth factor in decreasing wound-healing times by acting as a chemotactic agent and mitogen for fibroblasts, smooth muscle cells, and inflammatory cells. Transforming growth factor-beta (TGF-β) acts as a chemotactic agent for fibroblasts and macrophages, a mitogen for macrophages, smooth muscle cells, and osteoblasts. It has an inhibitory effect on endothelial cells, various epithelial cell types, and lymphocytes. Transforming growth factor-alpha (TGF-α) is a potent angiogenesis factor. Epidermal growth factor is a potent chemotactic and mitogenic agent for keratinocytes and fibroblasts. Fibroblast growth factor is mitogenic for mesenchymal cells and endothelial cells and stimulates keratinocytes. Keratinocyte growth factor is a highly specific mitogen for keratinocytes and stimulates migration of keratinocytes. Insulin-like growth factor stimulates the synthesis of glycogen, protein, and glycosaminoglycans. It will also increase collagen synthesis by fibroblasts.

♥ It is quite possible that a combination of growth factors will be more beneficial than any single growth factor. Some studies investigating specific growth factors have not shown as positive effects as growth factor "soup." Further studies will need to be performed to accurately determine the role of exogenous growth factors in equine wound healing.

☞ In all likelihood the growth factors will have the greatest benefit in the granulating and epithelialization stages of wound-healing and will be used with other synthetic dressings.

Semi-Occlusive Foam Dressings ⊙

✓ Foam dressings are semi-occlusive dressings for use on mildly exudative wounds (Figure 6-28).

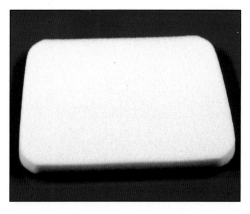

Figure 6-28 Semi-occlusive foam dressing (Hydrasorb™ Tyco Healthcare/Kendall).

🖐 They are generally used after healthy granulation tissue has formed and gross necrotic tissue and infection have been removed.

🖐 The use of a foam dressing will provide both a moist wound environment and a consistent thermal environment improving epithelialization and minimizing granulation tissue formation.

🖐 If there is exuberant granulation tissue present, the excess tissue should be trimmed back prior to dressing application.

🖐 The foam dressings can be changed every 4 to 7 days, depending on exudate level.

Case Example ♥

Signalment and History: A 3-month-old intact female American Paint horse was presented with a long-term history of flexural deformity of the forelimbs. Two weeks prior to presentation, the foal was noted to have pressure sores over the dorsal aspect of the mid cannon bone through the skin, sub-cutaneous tissue, and extensor tendon down to the level of the cannon bone.

Clinical Examination: On presentation, the filly was noted to have a wound at approximately 10 cm distal to the carpus on the dorsal aspect of the cannon bone through the skin, subcutaneous tissue, and extensor tendon. The region around the wound was swollen, and the filly was painful to palpation. Radiographs of the metacarpal region showed a periosteal response but no sequestrum. The leg was bandaged with a non-adherent pad with roll gauze and a standard pressure bandage with combine cotton. The bandage was changed every 2 to 3 days with steroid cream beginning at day 5 after presentation.

Ten days after presentation, the wound was noted to have mild exuberant granulation tissue, but had not changed significantly in size. At this time, the wound was cleaned with saline and a semi-occlusive foam pad (Hydrasorb™, Tyco Healthcare/Kendall) was secured directly to the wound surface with roll gauze and a pressure bandage (Figure 6-29).

When the bandage was removed on day 20, the wound had begun to epithelialize in from the wound edges, especially at the proximal aspect of the wound (Figure 6-30). The wound was cleaned with a surfactant-based wound cleanser and rinsed with saline. Another foam pad was placed over the wound and a pressure bandage applied.

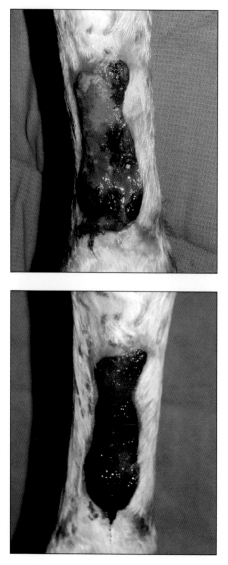

Figure 6-29 Distal cannon wound just prior to application of the first semi-occlusive foam dressing.

Figure 6-30 Wound at second bandage change, day 10 foam therapy.

The bandage was again changed on day 23 with continued epithelialization. On day 27, there was no exuberant granulation tissue present and the wound had continued to epithelialize (Figure 6-31). The wound was again covered with a foam dressing and left in place for 5 days.

On day 36, the wrap was removed and the wound size had continued to decrease. The wound area was now noted to be approximately 60% that of day 10 when the foam dressings were first applied (Figure 6-32).

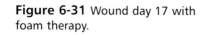

Figure 6-31 Wound day 17 with foam therapy.

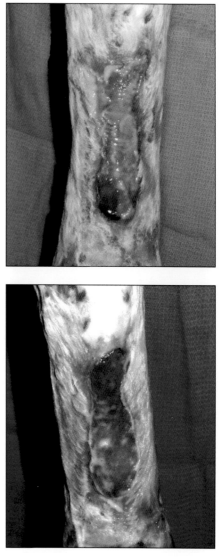

Figure 6-32 Wound day 26 with foam therapy.

By day 40, the wound had continued to contract and epithelialize (Table 6-8). At this time, the wound was rebandaged with a foam dressing and care transferred to a different veterinarian. Wound care for the next 36 days included a non-adherent dressing with and/or without a steroid cream.

Table 6-8
Wound Types for Semi-Occlusive Foam Dressings

Mildly exudative wounds
Clean wounds with healthy granulation tissue
Wounds with mildly exuberant granulation tissue

The foal re-presented 76 days after the initial presentation. The wound now had exuberant granulation tissue at the most proximal and distal extent of the wound where the wound had been treated with a steroid cream. The wound dimensions at these areas had not changed since the last picture 42 days previously. The wound had continued to contract in the middle where the granulation tissue had not become exuberant and no steroid cream had been applied (Figure 6-33). The use of steroids has been shown to reduce not only granulation tissue formation but epithelialization as well. See the following section on steroids for a more in-depth discussion. It is possible that the wound would have healed by this time if a semi-occlusive foam dressing had been continued.

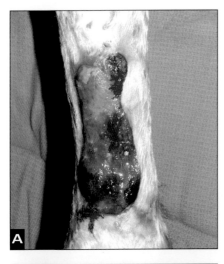

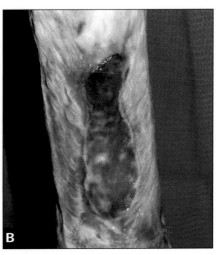

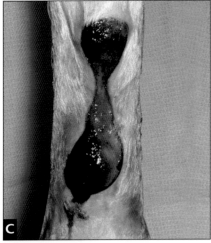

Figure 6-33 Wound showing comparisons. **A.** Day 0 foam therapy. **B.** Day 26 foam therapy. **C.** Cessation of foam therapy after 40 days.

Steroids

✓ Steroids have long been a mainstay in equine wound care for the reduction of granulation tissue. They are typically used to inhibit or reduce the volume of exuberant granulation tissue (Figure 6-34).

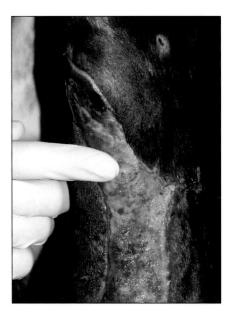

Figure 6-34 Application of a steroid cream.

☞ In vitro studies have shown that hydrocortisone up-regulates plasminogen activator inhibitor-1 and down-regulates plasminogen activators. The plasminogen activators play an important role in wound homeostasis. This change likely inhibits proteolytic matrix degradation and re-epithelialization, which are both necessary for rapid and efficient wound repair. Dexamethasone has been shown to interfere with the synthesis and degradation of both type I and III collagen in rats. Type III collagen has a major role in the induction of wound healing and is affected more dramatically by dexamethazone. Triamcinalone has been shown to decrease vascular growth and consequently granulation tissue formation in rabbits. Topical administration was more severe in reducing angiogenesis than was systemic therapy. Testosterone has been shown to delay wound healing in mice.

✋ At this time, it is not advisable to use steroids during wound healing if effective cosmetic wound healing is desired.

131

☝ Excess granulation tissue should be removed by surgical methods and moist wound healing techniques used to improve wound healing without excess granulation tissue.

Summary

♥ In summary, the advantages of moist healing include prevention of wound desiccation, increased re-epithelialization rate, prevention of eschar formation, decreased inflammation, enhanced autolytic debridement, a bacterial barrier and subsequent decreased rate of infection with occlusive dressings, and cost efficiency. There are many options available for treating wounds, each with benefits at certain stages of healing. The author has had the most experience using five main dressing types including hypertonic saline, antimicrobial dressings, hydragels, calcium alginate dressings, and semi-occlusive foam dressings. Clinical judgment will help the clinician determine which dressing to use at each stage of the treatment process. See table 6-9 for a partial listing of suture manufacturers.

☝ The following table and flow chart will give a perspective on how the author decides which dressing to use (Figures 6-35 and 6-36).

Table 6-9
Partial Listing Of Dressing Manufactures

MANUFACTURER	DRESSING TYPE
Tyco Healthcare/Kendall	Curasalt, Kerlix A.M.D. Curafil, Curagel, Curasorb, Hydrasorb, Expandover II
MacLeod	Intracell: Maltrodextran
Acell Inc	Acell Vet
PRN Pharmaceutical	Collasate
The Franklin-Williams Company	CombiRoll
3M	Gamgee, Vet Wrap, Elastacon

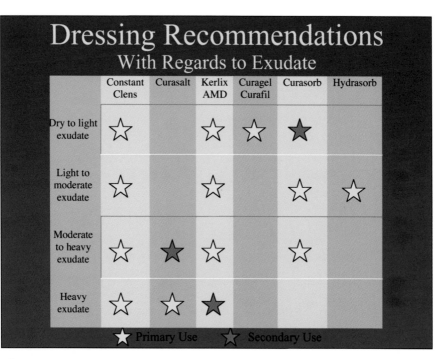

Figure 6-35 Wound care selection table with regards to exudate level.

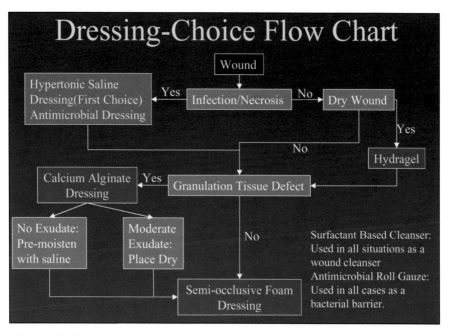

Figure 6-36 Flow chart showing wound care dressing selection.

Caustic Agents

✓ Caustic agents have been used in wound healing both to encourage and retard excess granulation tissue.

✋ While these agents have been used on wounds that have successfully healed, they should be avoided because there are better methods available.

Excess Granulation Tissue

✓ Excess or exuberant granulation tissue is a common problem in equine wounds left to heal by second intention.

☞ Whenever the granulation tissue grows beyond or is proud to the skin, it will slow the process of epithelialization. When this happens, wound healing will often come to a standstill.

✓ Many techniques have been used to reduce exuberant granulation tissue including sharp debridement, caustic agents, steroid cream, and more recently, semi-occlusive foam dressings.

☞ Sharp debridement is still the method of choice for granulation tissue removal (Figure 6-37).

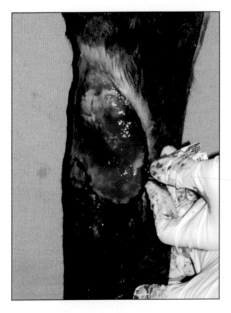

Figure 6-37 Sharp debridement of granulation tissue.

✓ The use of a tourniquet may allow the practitioner better visualization of the tissue being removed. Because granulation tissue has a very poor nerve supply, it is generally possible to remove the granulation tissue without need for local anesthetic. If undermining of the skin edge is necessary, local anesthetic should be used.

✋ Caustic agents, while effective in removing granulation tissue, are too harmful to the rest of the tissue and should not be used.

✓ If minimal exuberant granulation tissue is present, semi-occlusive foam dressings have proven beneficial in reducing granulation tissue. However, the most effective way to remove granulation tissue is to sharply debride it.

⌐ A good pressure bandage should be placed over the debrided wound and left in place for 1 to 2 days. The author prefers to use a semi-occlusive foam dressing (Figure 6-38).

♥ It is the author's observation that exuberant granulation tissue is less of a problem if moist wound-healing concepts are strictly followed.

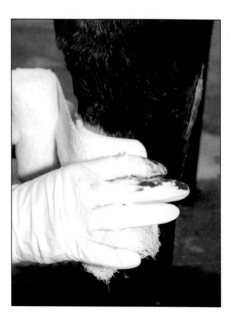

Figure 6-38
Application of a semi-occlusive foam dressing after surgical debridement of exuberant granulation tissue.

Non-Healing Wounds

☞ When a wound does not heal in a reasonable amount of time, it is important to rule out the underlying cause.

✋ Infection and/or the presence of foreign material are some of the most common reasons for retarded healing in the horse.

✓ The author has been presented with multiple wounds that have had a very protracted healing time. In one case, a horse was presented to the ophthalmology section for a corneal ulcer. On physical examination it was noted that the entire cornea was edematous, and there was a large wound caudal to the orbit with necrotic debris exuding from the wound stoma. On further examination, a portion of a tree branch was identified and removed from the wound. The branch had been present for approximately 3 weeks. The horse lost the eye and was eventually euthanatized as the massater muscle sloughed. While there are no guarantees, it is possible that this horse would have been successfully treated with early removal of the foreign body. Thorough exploration of the wound using an instrument for a probe or ultrasound would have been useful in finding the wood.

✓ Other common findings in non-healing wounds are plant fibers such as grass awns. Once deep-seated infection is established, it is very difficult to find all of the foreign material and remove it from the wound.

☞ Hence, it is important to address the presence of foreign material as soon as possible to ease removal.

✓ Bone sequestra are another common finding that lead to prolonged wound healing. When equine bone is exposed to the air, such as with a dorsal canon bone laceration, bone sequestra may develop. When lacerations over the dorsal cannon bone occur, it is important to check the wound in approximately 2 weeks to determine if a sequestrum is present. Intermediate therapy using a moistened calcium alginate dressing may reduce sequestrum formation. The most effective way to do this is with a radiograph. Other common sources of sequestra are open fractures where bone fragments are left in the wound.

☞ Once the bone has become avascular, it is difficult for the body to resorb the bone and reduce the risk of infection.

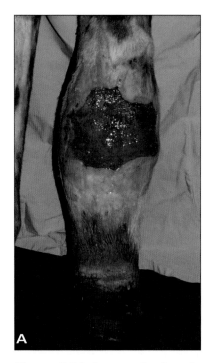 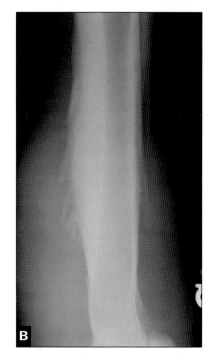

Figure 6-39 A. A non-healing chronic leg wound. **B.** Radiograph of the leg.

✓ In some cases, deep-seated bone infection without the presence of sequestra can occur and prolong wound healing (Figure 6-39). Long-term antibiotics are often necessary to remove the bacterial infection.

♥ Regardless of the cause, it is imperative to remove the source of infection to allow unimpeded wound healing. Radiographs, ultrasound, and wound exploration are the most common methods of finding foreign bodies. In certain cases, CT scans or MRI could be useful, but can only be performed on the head and extremities (see Section 3, Wound Exploration).

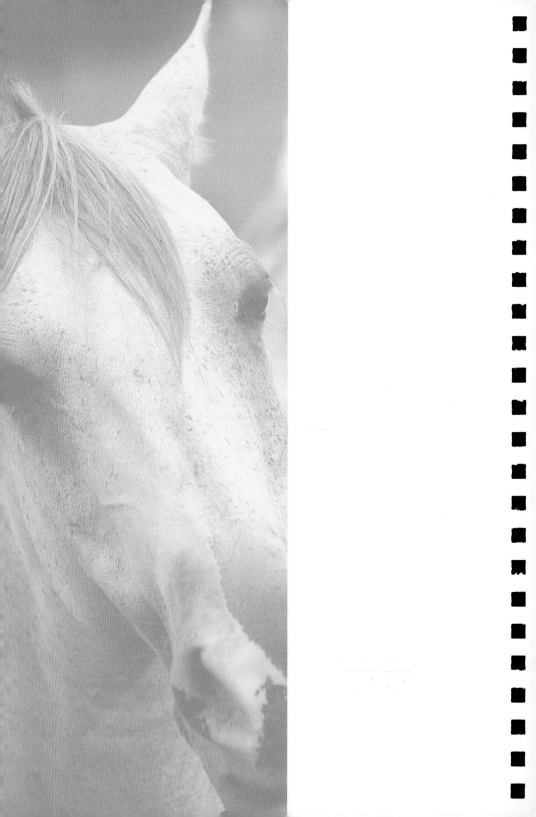

Section 7

Skin Grafting

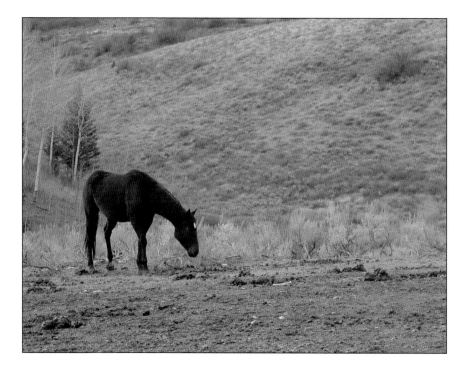

This section will help the practitioner to understand the principles of skin grafting. Common techniques and pitfalls will be discussed.

✓ Skin grafting can be a very useful tool in the armamentarium of the equine practitioner.

☞ Skin grafts not only cover granulation tissue and result in a more cosmetic end result, but they have also been shown to encourage wound contraction and epithelialization while decreasing exuberant granulation tissue.

✓ In most instances, wound healing can proceed effectively using the principles of second-intention healing. However, there are times when second-intention healing will not provide a cosmetic end result, or when the clients wish to speed the healing process. In these instances, the practitioner should consider performing skin grafts.

☞ Skin grafting in itself is not a difficult procedure.

✋ Most of the effort involves appropriate preparation of the wound bed and skin graft prior to placement and effective immobilization of the grafted area after skin graft placement (Table 7-1).

Table 7-1
Indications for Skin Grafting

Wounds that don't heal by contraction and epithelialization

Wounds where the cosmetic outcome is very important

Wounds where the client does not want to spend the time necessary for second-intention healing

Very large wounds

Immediate Wound Care

✋ Appropriate immediate wound care will provide the best substrate for not only wound healing but for eventual skin grafting.

✓ Skin grafts can be placed immediately after excision of skin masses or after appropriate wound care and second-intention wound healing has occurred.

☞ Following moist wound-healing principles will provide the practitioner with the most rapidly formed and best foundation for skin grafting.

☞ Effective wound debridement is always the most important first step in wound care. A wound that is free of bacteria and necrotic debris will begin healing more quickly than a wound with a large number of bacteria and mass of necrotic debris. See Section 2, Wound Preparation, Cleaning, and Debridement for more information on immediate wound care.

Bed Preparation

✓ As described above, preparation of the recipient bed for skin grafting really begins the day the wound is first examined.

⚡ Ideally the wound will be adequately debrided to remove necrotic debris and decrease bacterial numbers. After the wound has been adequately debrided and healthy granulation tissue is present, the wound will often be covered by a calcium alginate dressing to encourage granulation tissue formation up to the level of the surrounding skin edge.

⚡ Once granulation tissue has filled in the wound defect, a semi-occlusive foam dressing can be used. As soon as a normal pink granulation tissue bed is present, the wound can be grafted.

💣 It is critical that the practitioner not place a graft onto a bed of unhealthy or infected granulation tissue. It is always better to wait until the bed is healthy before performing a skin graft (Figure 7-1).

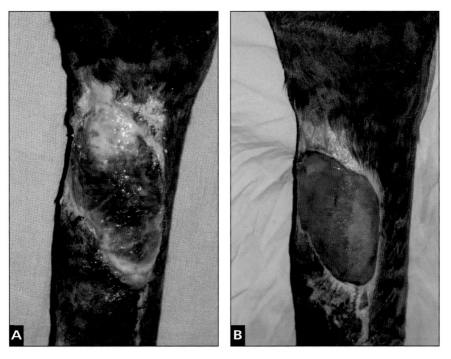

Figure 7-1 Granulation tissue beds. **A**. Unhealthy granulation tissue bed.
B. Healthy granulation tissue bed.

Types of Grafts

✓ There are three main types of skin grafts used in horses (Table 7-2). **Autografts** are the most commonly used grafts in equine wound care. They are cost effective and offer the lowest immune response of any grafts types. **Allografts** and **xenografts** are typically used to cover wounds temporarily. They have been found to decrease fluid loss, create a moist wound environment, and encourage healthy granulation bed formation. In this fashion, allografts and xenografts work similarly to semi-occlusive dressings. Allografts are harvested from cadavers that have been recently euthanized and are stored frozen. Xenografts are typically collected from pigs and are commercially available from several sources.

✓ If large areas of the body are affected, the use of allografts may be more cost effective than using semi-occlusive dressings, but proper preparation and storage is necessary to minimize bacterial infection.

Table 7-2
Types of Skin Grafts

Autografts	donor and recipient are the same animal
Allografts	donor and recipient are different animals but are of the same species
Xenografts	donor and recipient are from different species

Healing Stages of Skin Grafts

🗝 Adherence – Day 1. Before any other healing stages can occur, the graft must adhere to the wound bed. This bond is generally created by fibrin between the graft and the wound bed. This bond keeps the graft in close proximity to the wound bed allowing minimal distance for nutrients and blood vessels to travel. The fibrin will also act as a scaffold for migration of fibroblasts and endothelial cells. Successful adherence will allow the progression of the other stages of graft healing. If infection or excess movement is present, breakdown of the fibrin can be quite rapid leading to disruption of the fibrin bond and, consequently, adherence of the graft. Graft failure will result.

🗝 Plasmic Imbibition – Days 1-4. Graft nutrition is accomplished by plasmic imbibition until new blood vessels form. The blood vessels in the graft undergo vasospasm immediately after harvest. When the graft is placed on the recipient bed, the vessels relax allowing passive uptake of nutrients from the serum in the fibrin network between the graft and the recipient bed. Imbibition of serum will not provide enough nutrients or oxygen to keep a graft alive without revascularization. Cyanosis is expected in the early stages of graft healing, since the fluid does not really circulate through the graft. Excess movement or infection will minimize imbibition, leading to graft failure.

⚘ Revascularization – Days 3-7. Revascularization occurs by at least three different methods. Inosculation occurs when vessels in the graft anastomose with vessels in the recipient bed and is the most rapid method of revascularization. Another method is when capillary buds penetrate from the recipient bed into the graft vessels, using them as a conduit to revascularize the graft. Finally, capillary buds may penetrate the graft in areas other than old vessels to revascularize the graft. This is the slowest method of revascularization, since the growth rate of capillary buds is approximately 1 mm/day. Ideally the majority of revascularization will occur by inosculation which can occur in the first 2 days after grafting. Close proximity of the graft to the recipient bed is critical for sufficient inosculation to occur. The greater the distance between the graft and the recipient bed, the more likely that capillary buds will have to form an entirely new vascular network, and the greater likelihood of graft failure.

⚘ Final Organization. While fibrin is initially responsible for graft adherence, collagen is necessary to hold the graft permanently in place. Fibroblasts migrate into the space between the graft and the recipient bed using the fibrin as a scaffold. The collagen fibers and neovascularization provide a firm attachment of the graft to the recipient bed within 9 days of grafting.

Skin Graft Types

✓ Skin grafts are classified according to their thickness, shape, and source of tissue.

✓ Full-thickness grafts are composed of both the dermis and epidermis.

✓ Partial-thickness grafts are composed of the epidermis and part of the dermis.

⚘ Both full-thickness and partial-thickness grafts can be used in horses. Full-thickness grafts tend to give more cosmetic end results but are more difficult to apply successfully. Partial-thickness grafts tend to have a better success rate but have a less cosmetic end result.

✓ Small pieces of skin that are used as grafts are called pinch or punch grafts. Long strips of skin that are buried under the surface of the skin are called tunnel grafts. Large sheets of skin are called sheet grafts. Sheet grafts that are fenestrated are called mesh grafts.

☞ Non-meshed sheet grafts will generally provide the best cosmetic end result, but are the most likely to fail.

✓ Grafts that have a specific blood supply are called pedicle grafts. Pedicle grafts can be transferred locally without disrupting the vasculature or can be removed and transplanted to a distant site. When transferred to a distant site they are called free pedicle grafts, and are revascularized with microsurgical anastomotic techniques.

Grafting Techniques ⊙

✓ Just as there are different types of grafts, there are many techniques available for skin grafting.

✋ Each technique offers benefits and consequences, so the practitioner must be familiar with the different techniques to provide the best possible outcome for the patient and client.

✓ Grafts can either be harvested manually or by using motorized equipment. Harvesting by manual techniques has the obvious benefit of providing skin for grafting with minimal expense for necessary equipment. Motorized equipment, on the other hand, will generally provide a more consistent skin thickness and consequently a better chance for graft "take." As always, the pros and cons of each technique must be evaluated to maximize results for the patient and client.

☞ Whatever the method for grafting, the grafted tissue must have adequate capillary exposure to allow in-growth of blood vessels.

☞ The recipient bed must have an adequate granulation tissue bed without bacterial infection and with adequate capillary support for the graft.

☞ The practitioner must provide protection from mechanical disruption, hematoma formation, and infection.

♥ As soon as the graft is harvested, it is a race between attachment and revascularization of the graft and graft degeneration and failure.

Skin Graft Donor Sites

✓ Skin grafts can be taken from any portion of the horse.

💣 It is important to remember that wherever the skin graft is removed from disfigurement or scarring may result. For this reason, the ventral abdomen (Figure 7-2) or the neck under the mane (Figure 7-3) are the most common sites used to harvest skin grafts.

🔑 If possible, it is beneficial for cosmetic purposes to harvest the skin in an area that has similar color to the recipient bed.

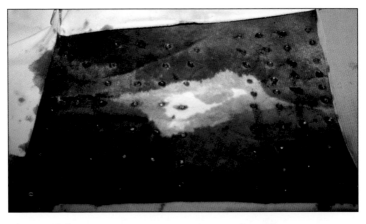

Figure 7-2 Abdominal donor site for punch grafts.

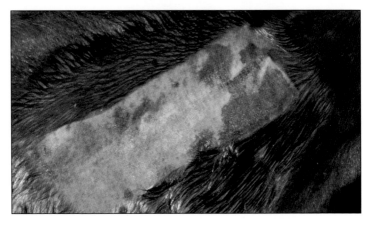

Figure 7-3 Neck donor site for pinch or punch grafts.

Animal Positioning, Anesthesia, and Sedation

✓ Skin grafting can be performed with the horse in a standing position while sedated (Figure 7-4) or in a recumbent position while anesthetized (Figure 7-5).

✓ To perform skin grafting on standing horses, it is best to sedate the horses adequately to reduce movement. While local anesthesia is not necessary for the recipient site, it is very important to perform at the skin-donor site. The author prefers to use a combination of detomidine and butorphanol for sedation.

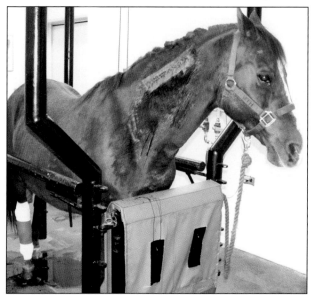

Figure 7-4 Standing horse undergoing skin graft procedure.

🗝 Obvious benefits of performing grafting on standing horses include elimination of special equipment for general anesthesia and reduced cost of the procedure. One less obvious benefit of performing skin grafts on standing horses is that the horse does not need to recover from anesthesia, and consequently will have less movement at the graft site. In many cases, as horses recover from general anesthesia, they will disrupt their dressings. The main downside to performing skin grafts on standing horses is animal movement and subsequent dislodging of the skin grafts during graft placement.

The main benefit to anesthetizing the horse prior to skin grafting is that the horse can be placed in whatever position is best for the surgeon to perform the harvesting and implantation of the graft. It is easy to place the grafts without the concerns of animal movement and dislodging of the graft. General anesthesia is usually necessary for performing sheet grafting.

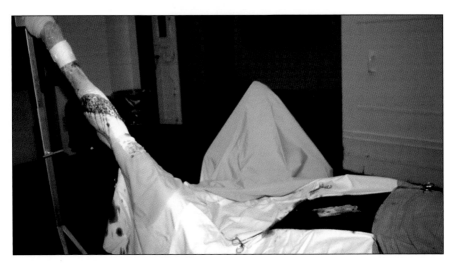

Figure 7-5 Horse in dorsal recumbency while under general anesthesia during skin graft procedure.

Pinch Grafting

✓ Pinch grafting can be performed on a standing horse using sedation and local anesthesia or in horses under general anesthesia.

✓ In the standing horse, the grafts are generally harvested from the neck.

It is important to select the side of the neck that the mane falls toward to minimize potentially unsightly scars.

The mane should be braided or taped and moved to the opposite side of the neck. The donor site should be clipped and local anesthetic infiltrated in an inverted "L" fashion to desensitize the area (Figure 7-3). If possible, the sub-cutaneous tissue deep to the donor skin should not be directly infiltrated. This will make removal of the sub-cutaneous tissues and fascia easier. The skin is generally tented with a tissue forceps or a needle, and the pinch of skin is excised with a scalpel blade (Figure 7-6).

147

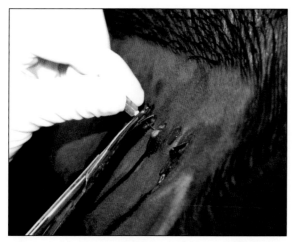

Figure 7-6
Use of a needle to elevate skin graft.

The size of the graft should generally be about 7 mm x 7 mm. Recipient pockets are created using a number 15 or 11 scalpel blade. The blade is inserted from a proximal to distal direction at about a 30 degree angle into the granulation tissue. The pockets are made approximately the same size as the skin grafts (Figure 7-7). Some practitioners will create pockets for the skin grafts in the granulation tissue of the recipient bed prior to harvesting the skin grafts.

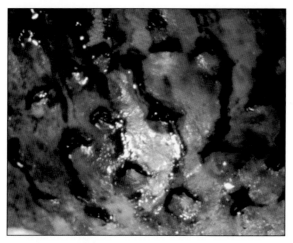

Figure 7-7
Pockets within the granulation tissue with pinch grafts in place.

The author prefers to harvest skin grafts first, place them on a blood or saline-soaked gauze (Figure 7-8), then make the recipient pockets and place the grafts. Using this method, grafts can be placed sequentially and rapidly, reducing the likelihood of graft displacement with animal movement. It will provide a better cosmetic end result if the grafts are placed so the hair grows in the same direction as the recipient area. This requires that the grafts be placed in the same orientation on the gauze before implantation.

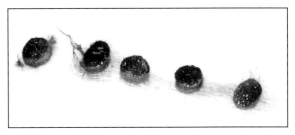

Figure 7-8 Punch grafts on saline soaked gauze.

The grafted area is covered with a semi-occlusive foam dressing that is held in place by an antimicrobial gauze (Kerlix A.M.D.™, Tyco Healthcare/Kendall) (Figure 7-9).

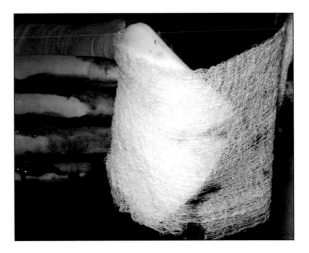

Figure 7-9
Semi-occlusive foam dressing over recipient bed being covered with antimicrobial roll gauze.

Next an elastic adhesive dressing is placed to maintain effective pressure at the dressing site and reduce dressing slippage. A standard pressure bandage (Figure 7-10) or cast is applied to minimize movement at the graft site. The donor sites are closed with interrupted sutures using a small absorbable suture material (Figure 7-11).

✓ In the anesthetized horse, the same procedure is followed except the grafts are generally harvested from the ventral abdomen of the horse. Local anesthetic is not required to desensitize the graft donor area.

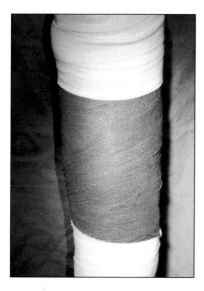

Figure 7-10 Pressure bandage over skin graft area.

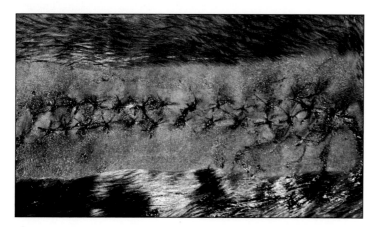

Figure 7-11 Neck showing closure of skin graft donor sites.

When making the recipient pockets in the granulation tissue, it is important to have the opening proximal and the deep portion of the pocket distal. This will reduce the possibility of the graft becoming dislodged and falling out of the pocket (Figure 7-12).

✓ The dressing technique is the same as previously described.

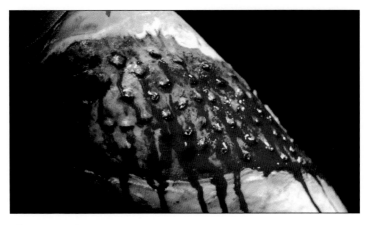

Figure 7-12 Pinch grafts in granulation recipient pockets. Note that the deep portion of the pocket is oriented distally. The horse is in dorsal recumbency with the leg pointing up.

Punch Grafting

✓ The technique for punch grafting is very similar to that of pinch grafting.

⚷ The main difference is that skin biopsy punches are used to create the skin grafts and the recipient pockets in the granulation tissue of the recipient bed. The author generally uses an 8 mm biopsy punch for the skin graft (Figure 7-13) and a 6 mm punch for the recipient pocket (Figure 7-14).

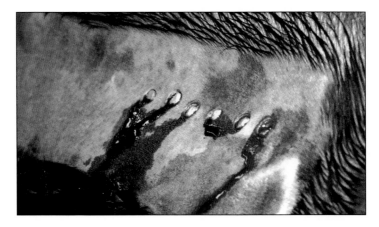

Figure 7-13 Punch grafts within the donor site on the neck.

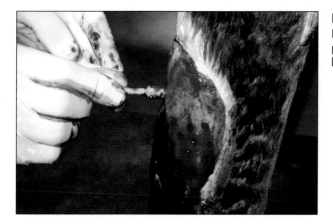

Figure 7-14
Making recipient pockets in the granulation tissue.

🖐 When using biopsy punches, it is easy to include excess sub-cutaneous and fascial tissue with the donor skin. Sub-cutaneous tissue should be removed from the deep aspect of the skin graft to provide access to the capillaries for imbibition and revascularization.

✓ It is possible to use a scalpel blade to make recipient pockets like those described for pinch grafting.

🖐 The main advantage of using a punch biopsy tool in the recipient bed is that the graft is never covered by granulation tissue and spreading of epithelial cells is more rapid. The main disadvantage is that blood or serum can build behind the grafts and push them out, leading to graft failure (Figure 7-15).

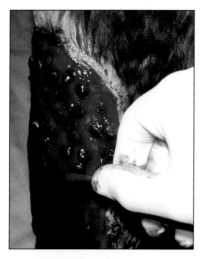

Figure 7-15 Seating punch grafts with a cotton-tipped applicator.

✓ Punch grafting will often have a slight cosmetic benefit over pinch grafts at the donor site. The dressing technique is the same as previously described for pinch grafting. Epithelialization spreads from the islands of graft tissue to cover the wound. In many cases wound contraction is stimulated by grafting (Figure 7-16).

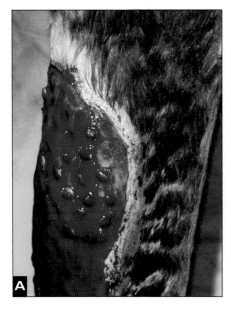

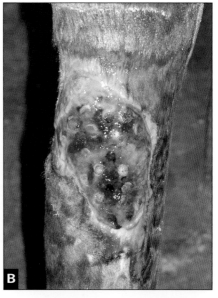

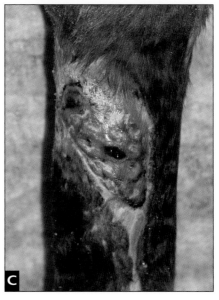

Figure 7-16 Skin graft.
A. Immediately upon completion.
B. Day 7 at first bandage change.
C. Day 60.

Tunnel Grafting

✔ Tunnel grafts are composed of long lengths of full-thickness skin 2-3 mm wide which can be harvested from anywhere on the axial portion of the body.

☞ The strips are removed by making parallel incisions 2-3 mm apart through the skin into the sub-cutaneous tissue. The strips are removed from the skin with a scalpel blade to minimize the amount of sub-cutaneous tissue and fascia. The strips are cut just long enough to allow enough extra skin to suture the grafts at each end of the tunnel. An alligator forceps is used to tunnel through the granulation tissue 5 to 6 mm deep to the surface and grasp the strip of skin. Grafts are placed approximately 2 cm apart.

✋ The practitioner must be careful to keep the epidermis positioned superficially.

✔ The ends of the graft are secured with an interrupted suture (Figure 7-17). Six to 10 days after grafting, the overlying granulation tissue and the granulation tissue between the grafts is surgically removed.

☞ The benefit of tunnel grafting is that more skin is placed in the graft than with pinch or punch grafts, yet they require less specialized equipment than is necessary with sheet grafts.

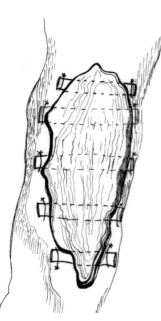

Figure 7-17 The application of tunnel grafts.

☙ Tunnel grafts are not as subject to movement as other grafts since they are buried in the granulation tissue. This makes them a good choice in areas such as the hock where excess movement is common.

Mesh Grafting

✓ Non-meshed sheet grafts are very rarely used in equine skin grafting.

✓ The volume of skin required, along with the reduced probability of graft "take," make meshed sheet grafts much more common.

☙ Horses should be anesthetized prior to sheet grafting.

♥ Meshed-sheet grafts will generally provide a more cosmetic end result than will the pinch, punch, or tunnel grafts. However, the large amount of skin removed may cause a more severe cosmetic blemish at the donor site. It is therefore important to select the donor site carefully. The most common donor site is the ventral abdomen or the pectoral region (Figure 7-18)

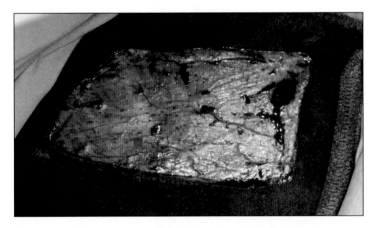

Figure 7-18 Sheet graft donor site - the ventral abdomen.

💣 Grafts should not be harvested in the girth area.

✓ Sheet grafts can be harvested with a scalpel blade but it is generally best to harvest them with a dermatome (Figure 7-19). Used properly, a dermatome will provide the practitioner with a skin graft of even thickness. The cost associated with a dermatome and the difficulty in setting up the dermatome are often deterrents to their use. In most cases, the grafts will then be meshed to provide expansion of the graft and areas of fluid escape. Fenestration can be as easy as using a scalpel blade or as complicated as using a commercial mesher (Figure 7-20).

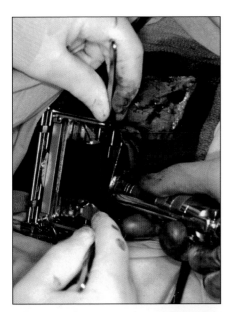

Figure 7-19 Dermatome harvesting a full-thickness sheet graft.

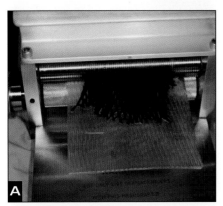

Figure 7-20
A. Picture of full-thickness skin graft in mesher. **B**. Meshed sheet graft.

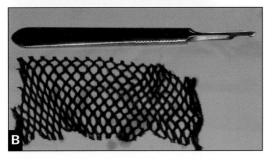

Commercial units will provide the most even fenestration and probably the best cosmetic end result. The graft is generally attached by placing several interrupted sutures between the graft and the surrounding skin (Figure 7-21).

✓ In many cases, more than one graft is harvested and stored in case the first graft does not take. Grafts can be stored for up to 4 weeks and sequentially applied while the horse is standing (Figure 7-22).

♥ Sheet grafts are the best choice when excising a skin mass and immediately placing a graft. Punch or pinch grafts are generally more commonly used due to the minimal equipment necessary and the ability to perform the technique in a standing horse.

Figure 7-21 Mesh graft at recipient site.

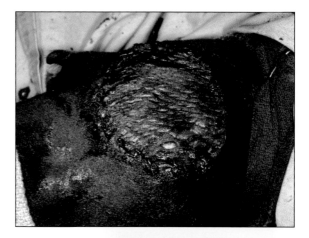

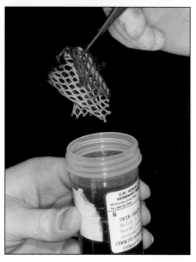

Figure 7-22
Placing extra mesh graft in storage media.

Pedicle Grafting

✓ Pedicle grafts require general anesthesia.

✓ A full-thickness piece of skin is elevated from the donor site. If the main vascular supply is left intact, it is an anchored pedicle graft; if the main vascular supply is transected for transfer to a distal site, it is a free-pedicle graft.

🖐 Pedicle grafts require a thorough understanding of the vascular supply. Free pedicle grafts require specialized equipment such as operating microscopes for reattachment of the graft. This type of grafting will not be covered in this book.

Grafting Aftercare

Dressing Choices

✓ Many dressing types have been used to cover skin grafts.

♥ The ideal dressing should provide a secure environment with no motion and no bacterial penetration. At the same time the dressing will need to provide management of wound exudate by maintaining a moist wound environment and evacuation of excess exudate if necessary.

🔑 The dressing should not adhere to the graft or the recipient bed to reduce the chance of dislodging the graft during dressing changes.

✓ Petrolatum impregnated dressings have often been considered a mainstay in covering skin graft sites. Typical non-adherent dressings can successfully minimize graft adherence to the dressings but often do not do an adequate job of managing exudate.

✓ Newer semi-occlusive foam dressings are very useful in skin grafting (Figure 7-9). They provide the practitioner with a dressing that has the previously described necessary characteristics.

🖐 In most cases, by the time a skin graft is placed, there will not be an excessive amount of exudate. For this reason, it is important to use a primary dressing that will not dry out the recipient bed.

✓ It is also important to select the appropriate secondary dressing to ensure the best chance for success in skin grafting. A dressing that provides an antimicrobial barrier can be very beneficial (Figure 7-9).

Frequency of Dressing Changes

✓ Frequent dressing changes have the benefit of allowing regular observation of the graft site. During this observation, it is possible to reduce or remove any serum or hematoma pockets that may have developed between the graft and the recipient bed. It is also possible to determine if the graft is viable or if it has died. However, it has been shown that graft viability can be difficult to determine for up to two weeks after graft implantation. Unfortunately, frequent dressing changes also provide an entry point for bacteria and possible dislodging of the graft.

✓ Less frequent or weekly dressing changes provide an environment with less motion at the graft site, reducing the possibility of dislodging the graft. Fewer bandage changes have been shown to reduce the chance of introducing bacteria into the wound. The practitioner will have to weigh the positive and negative aspects associated with each of the bandage changing frequencies and use the best frequency for the wound presented.

⌐ The author chooses to leave the first bandage on for one week and then change the dressings as needed.

Wound Immobilization ◉

✓ Immobilization of the graft requires appropriate dressing choices and cooperation by the patient. Since achieving patient cooperation with horses is difficult at best, appropriate dressing selection along with coaptation may be beneficial in preventing grafts from dislodging.

⌐ Appropriate graft suturing can be helpful when using sheet grafts.

⌐ A firm pressure bandage should be placed over all grafted areas (Figure 7-23). Bulky bandages have a greater tendency to move than do less bulky bandages.

⌐ Cast application is often very helpful in immobilizing the grafted areas, especially when the grafted areas occur over mobile areas such as joints (Figure 7-24). Cast complications can occur, but this consequence is generally offset by the benefits of graft immobilization.

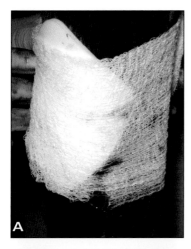

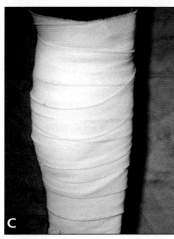

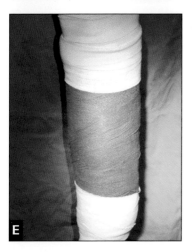

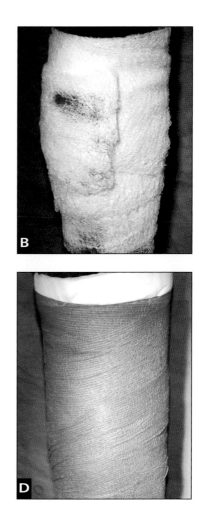

Figure 7-23
Dressings after grafting. **A**. Primary dressing of semi-occlusive foam. **B**. Secondary dressing of antimicrobial roll gauze. **C**. Elastic bandage to hold primary and secondary dressings in place. **D**. Combine cotton held in place with roll gauze and elastic wrap for pressure. **E**. Finished bandage.

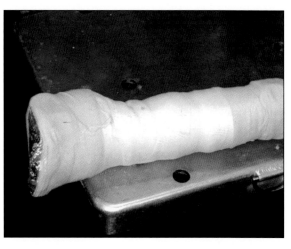

Figure 7-24 Cast applied after grafting a wound over the fetlock.

Reasons for Graft Failure

Inappropriate Type of Graft

✓ While sheet grafts will provide the best cosmetic end result, they are also the most difficult to work with.

☞ Using a sheet graft over a movable area such as a joint is likely to lead to graft failure.

☞ The use of punch or pinch grafts over very large skin defects will be helpful, but are not likely to provide enough skin to enhance cosmetic repair.

☞ Partial-thickness skin grafts are more likely to provide a successful outcome, since there are more capillaries available for imbibition and inosculation.

Inadequate Graft Preparation

☞ Inadequate removal of sub-cutaneous fat and fascia can reduce or inhibit revascularization.

✓ While hair follicle orientation is important to the cosmetic outcome, it will not affect the "take" of the graft.

Inadequate Recipient Bed Preparation

💣☀ The most appropriate bed for grafting is a young, healthy, pink, well vascularized bed of granulation tissue. Chronic, fibrous, infected, or poorly vascularized granulation tissue will not provide an acceptable recipient bed for grafting. These beds will have to be debrided and dressed to provide the best bed for grafting.

Infection

💣☀ Bacterial infection will stimulate fibrin breakdown, inhibit fibrin formation, and inhibit graft adherence. Accumulation of purulent debris will provide a layer of fluid and debris between the graft and the recipient bed which will slow or stop nutrition from flowing to the graft. It is difficult to predict bacterial numbers based upon granulation tissue appearance. Bacterial numbers greater that 10^6 per gram of tissue will generally lead to graft failure. Quantitative bacteriology is useful in determining the actual bacterial numbers. If granulation tissue looks healthy and still rejects the graft, it is important to perform quantitative cultures.

Separation of Graft from Wound Bed

💣☀ Any separation of the graft from the recipient bed can inhibit plasmic imbibition, and graft adherence, and delay revascularization leading to graft necrosis. Graft separation can be caused by fluid accumulation, improper tension, and/or movement. Fluid accumulation is typically only a problem in sheet grafts. Fluid can be removed by meshing the graft with either a machine or scalpel cuts. Fluid accumulation is also reduced with appropriate pressure bandages. Some surgeons suggest checking grafts daily to remove fluid accumulation under graft; others recommend not disturbing the graft for at least 7 days. Fluid accumulation is generally not considered a problem with punch, pinch, or tunnel grafts. However, it is important to remove the serum and clot in punch graft holes prior to graft placement.

Graft Movement

♦※ Graft movement is a common cause of graft failure. Movement will reduce graft adherence, consequently inhibiting plasmic imbibition, revascularization, and collagen formation between the graft and the recipient bed. Movement can be caused by placing the graft over a joint, or by using inappropriate dressings, or by infection or fluid accumulation. Choosing the appropriate dressings and including external coaptation in the form of a cast will reduce movement at the junction of the graft and recipient bed interface.

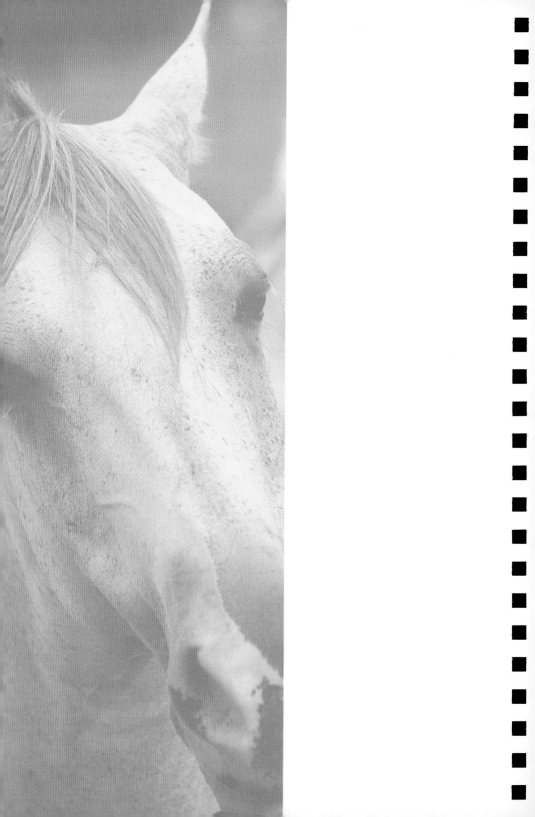

Section 8

Specific Wound
Considerations

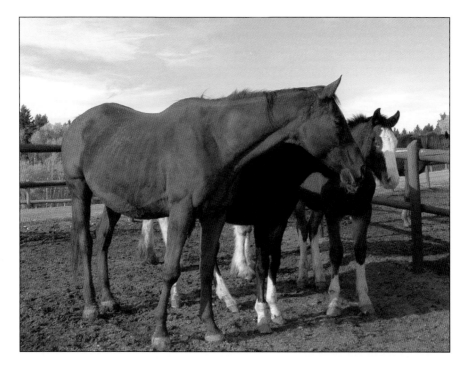

This section will cover specific wound considerations that offer special challenges to the practitioner.

Heel Bulb Lacerations/Hoof Wall Avulsions ◉

✓ Heel bulb lacerations occur frequently in equine practice and can involve anything from the skin to the coffin joint. In many cases, the wounds are grossly contaminated with dirt, manure, and/or bedding.

☞ The foot contains many vital structures whose involvement cannot be ruled out without a thorough and complete physical examination. When the digital arteries are involved in the laceration, blood loss can be quite spectacular.

✋ If the client is present during the case work-up, it is worthwhile to warn him or her that the wound will start bleeding again once cleaning begins.

✓ A basi-sesamoid or abaxial-sesamoid nerve block should be performed to allow a thorough examination. A sterile water soluble lubricating gel is placed in the wound to trap hair while the area surrounding the laceration is clipped. After clipping, the sterile gel is rinsed from the wound with a combination of sterile saline spray and woven gauze manipulation.

✋ Aseptic technique should be used until the practitioner is confident the wound does not involve the tendon sheath, the coffin joint, or the navicular bursa. The distal extent of the digital tendon sheath extends to near the heel bulb region.

✓ Povidone-iodine or chlorhexidine scrub can be used to clean the skin adjacent to the wound, but should not be used in the wound.

☞ The leg should be examined in both weight bearing (Figure 8-1) and non-weight bearing positions. In a non-weight bearing position, it is often possible to examine the wound more thoroughly and check for involvement of critical structures such as the digital tendon sheath, deep digital flexor tendon, navicular bursa, coffin joint, and/or the neurovascular bundle.

💣 If involvement of any of the synovial structures is suspected, the practitioner must rule them out by aseptically preparing a site distant to the laceration and injecting saline into the synovial space to look for leakage (Figure 8-2).

Figure 8-1
A heel bulb laceration. (Courtesy
of Dr. Troy Trumble)

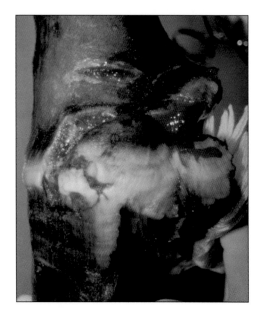

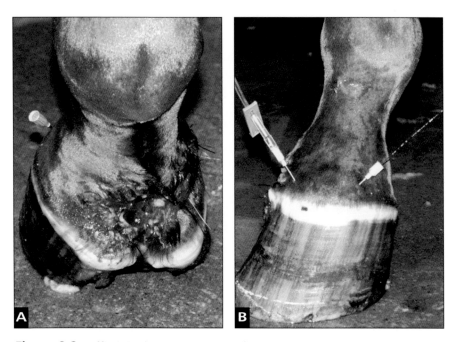

Figure 8-2 Coffin joint lavage. **A**. Wound from palmar aspect. **B**. Dorsal aspect
of leg showing coffin joint lavage.

✔ If there is no involvement, further intervention is straightforward. The wound is debrided as needed with either sharp or physical debridement. If possible, the skin is sutured to close the wound as much as possible.

☞ The amount of wound contamination will be the final determinant in closing the wound. If the wound is too contaminated, it should be treated with a hypertonic saline dressing and covered with an antimicrobial dressing. The dressings can be changed every 48 hours.

✔ When the wound is clean and appropriate debridement has been performed, the skin can be sutured.

✔ The wound should be covered with a semi-occlusive foam dressing held in place with antimicrobial roll gauze and the foot placed in a "slipper" cast.

✔ To apply a "slipper" cast, appropriate sized stockinet is chosen and placed over the foot up to the mid-cannon region. Cast felt is placed around the leg just distal to the fetlock joint. Approximately 3 rolls of 4-inch fiberglass cast material are rolled over the foot up to the top of the felt. The leg is held in a neutral non-weight bearing position until the cast has cured, then the horse is allowed to bear weight. The stockinet is rolled down over the cast and secured with an elastic bandage. An elastic bandage is placed from the cast to the skin to stop foreign material from entering the top of the cast. Rubber (car inner tube) can be placed over the bottom of the cast to improve traction and wear (Figure 8-3). The cast should be left in place for 2 to 3 weeks then removed.

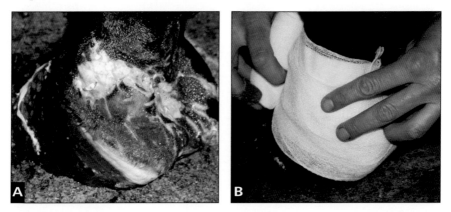

Figure 8-3 Application of a "slipper" cast. **A**. Heel bulb laceration. **B**. Applying semi-occlusive foam dressing and antimicrobial roll gauze. **C**. Application of stockinet. **D**. Felt just below the fetlock. **E**. Application of cast material. **F**. Foot on ground. **G**. Cast with rubber, duct tape, and elastic bandage.

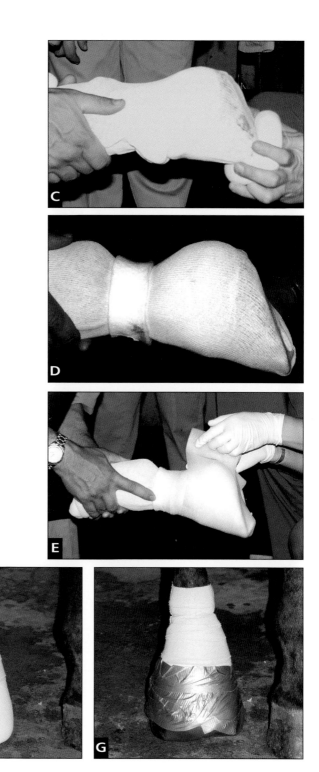

☞ There is a lot of skin movement in the hoof region that precludes good skin healing. A "slipper" cast will reduce the motion without predisposing the horse to cast sores (Figure 8-4).

♥ If there is synovial involvement, aggressive therapy involving synovial lavage, regional antibiotic perfusion, and systemic antibiotic therapy is instituted.

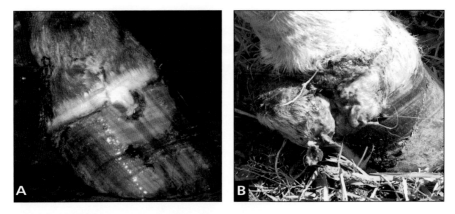

Figure 8-4 Heel bulb lacerations. **A**. Foot at 3 weeks after slipper cast application. **B**. Foot at 3 weeks that did not have a slipper cast applied.

☞ Region antibiotic perfusion involves placing a tourniquet in the mid-cannon region and injecting diluted antibiotics into one of the vascular structures (Figure 8-5). The author prefers to use an 18-gauge butterfly catheter. In most cases, an aminoglycoside such as amikacin (500 to 750 mg) or a cephalosporin such as cefazolin (1 gram) are used for the perfusion. It is possible to use one antibiotic for joint lavage and the other for regional perfusion, maximizing the antibiotic effect in the tissues. The antibiotics for the perfusion should be diluted with normal saline (35 to 60 ml). The tourniquet is left in place for 20 minutes, then removed.

☞ The wound is packed with a hypertonic saline dressing and covered with antimicrobial roll gauze (Figure 8-6). The synovial lavage and perfusion should be repeated 24 to 48 hours later and a similar dressing applied.

✓ As soon as the synovial membrane has sealed, a "slipper" cast should be applied as previously described.

✍ While casts can be applied without suturing the skin, the cosmetic result is generally better if the skin can be sutured. Delaying closure for up to 1 week is acceptable.

Figure 8-5 Leg with tourniquet after regional perfusion.

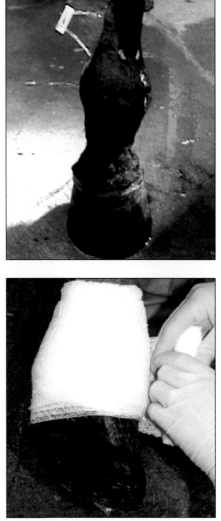

Figure 8-6 Application of hypertonic saline dressing and antimicrobial roll gauze.

💣 The owners should be warned that if the coronary band is involved, a hoof crack may develop.

✓ In some cases, horses can become lame when large scars develop at the heel bulb laceration site. The lameness seems to be associated with the disparate rigidity of the hoof wall, supple skin, and rigid scar. Application of vitamin E cream to soften the scar has obviated the lameness in some horses.

✓ Heel bulb avulsions are a challenging variation of heel bulb lacerations (Figure 8-7). A portion of hoof wall is lost with heel bulb avulsions.

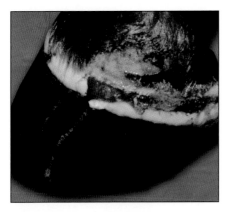

Figure 8-7 Hoof wall avulsion at presentation.

The initial work-up is identical to that of a heel bulb laceration. After all of the critical structures have been identified and all emergency therapy has been performed, the avulsion is addressed.

✔ It is important to identify how much of the hoof wall is involved and consequently how much will need to be removed. (Figure 8-8).

♥ It is not realistic to consider salvaging the avulsed wall and healing will progress more quickly with the avulsed tissue removed.

✔ If the laceration/avulsion involves the coronary band, it may be useful to try and suture the coronary-band tissue back to the leg as a type of graft. In many cases, the tissue will not adhere but it is worth the try because it can always be removed.

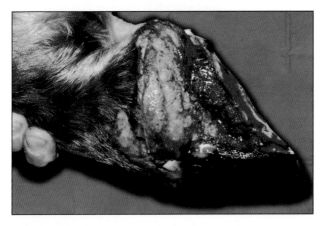

Figure 8-8 Foot with avulsed wall removed.

⚡ Foot support is best achieved using a bar shoe of some type (Figure 8-9).

✓ Local therapy will generally involve a hypertonic saline dressing covered by antimicrobial roll gauze and a pressure bandage. Once adequate debridement has occurred, a calcium alginate dressing is used. Eventually semi-occlusive foam dressings are used. If coronary-band reconstruction was attempted, a "slipper" cast should be applied.

✋ Acrylic may be placed over the hoof wall defect only after the deep tissue has cornified.

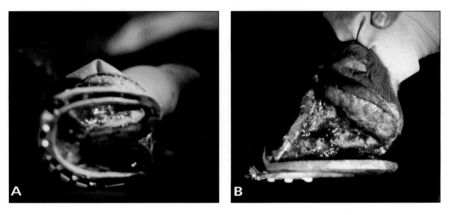

Figure 8-9 Hoof wall avulsion with heart-bar shoe. **A.** Solar view. **B.** Lateral view.

Lacerations of Synovial Structures ⊙

✋ There are many synovial structures in the horse including joints, tendon sheaths, and bursas.

♥ It is important to understand the anatomy of the horse well enough to know where these synovial structures are located (Figure 8-10). Whenever a laceration is close to one of these areas, it is critical to confirm or rule out synovial involvement. Infection of synovial structures can be very difficult to treat and increased time between injury and treatment will often lead to a worse prognosis. Early intervention, on the other hand, will often lead to a good to excellent prognosis.

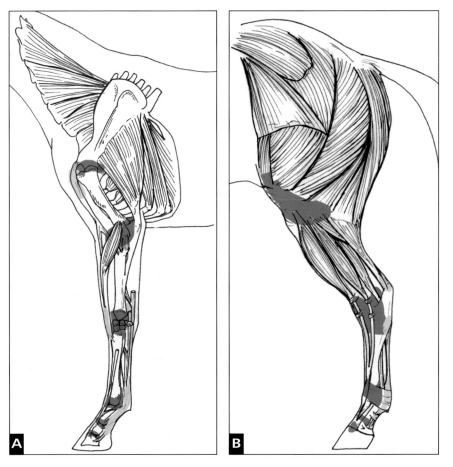

Figure 8-10 Drawing of **A**. front leg, and **B**. hind leg showing positions of common synovial structures. Orange highlights--joint capsules; yellow highlights--tendon sheaths.

♥ Consequently, the practitioner is responsible not only for performing a thorough examination, but also for educating their clients as to where important structures are. Then the clients will be more likely to get their animals treated in a more expedient manner.

✓ There are two main methods for confirming or ruling out synovial involvement. In either method, the leg must be clipped and prepared for exploration.

💣 Strict aseptic technique should be used to minimize the possibility of introducing bacterial contamination. Local anesthesia should be performed if possible because it allows the practitioner to examine the area more thoroughly.

✓ The easiest but least productive method is digital palpation.

🔓 Sterile gloves are donned and the area palpated. The leg should be palpated in a weight-bearing position as well as a non-weight bearing position. When the foot is off the ground, an assistant moves the leg through a range-of-motion exercise. The integrity of the medial and lateral collateral ligaments should be assessed at this time (Figure 8-11). Radiographs should be taken to rule out avulsion fractures.

♥ If an open synovial structure is confirmed, appropriate therapy should be instituted. If synovial involvement cannot be confirmed, synovial distension should be performed to rule out involvement.

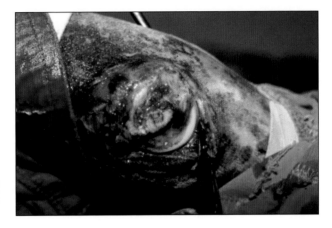

Figure 8-11 Fetlock with lateral collateral ligament disruption.

🔓 To perform synovial distention, the leg should be aseptically prepared to minimize bacterial introduction into the synovial structure.

♥ The entire procedure should be performed in an aseptic fashion.

🔓 The needle should be placed through the skin into the synovial structure from a site distant to the injury (Figure 8-12). In some cases, this can be almost impossible especially in long-standing wounds. Obviously, a good understanding of equine synovial anatomy is a must in these cases.

⬤ If the practitioner does not feel confident performing this procedure, adequate first aid should be initiated and the horse referred.

🔓 After the needle has been inserted, synovial fluid should be aspirated if at all possible. This sample should be split into two aliquots, one for cytology, and one for bacterial culture and sensitivity. In many

175

cases of synovial involvement, there will be minimal fluid left in the synovial cavity and no cytology can be performed. After attempting to collect synovial fluid, sterile saline is injected into the synovial structure. Generally a 20 to 60 ml syringe is chosen depending on the size of synovial space. If the saline injects easily and fluid exits the wound, synovial involvement is confirmed. If the saline injects easily yet no fluid exits the wound and there is no back-pressure, more saline should be injected. If ,while injecting the saline, the synovial structure distends and upon release of the plunger there is back flow into the syringe, the synovial structure is deemed intact.

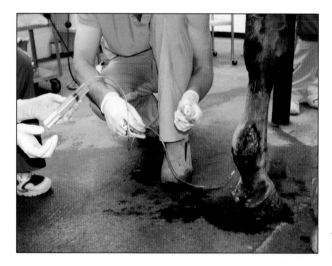

Figure 8-12 Digital tendon sheath showing synovial lavage.

In chronic wounds, it is possible that the synovial membrane will have sealed and will not communicate with the wound. In these cases, fluid collection for cytology is essential.

When it has been confirmed that the synovial structure is involved in the wound, appropriate therapy should be instituted. There are many options to treating contaminated or infected synovial structures. The most involved and, generally, best way to treat is anesthetizing the animal and performing an arthroscopic or tenoscopic evaluation and lavage. High volumes of fluid can be flushed through the joint or sheath, respectively, and any accumulated fibrin can be removed. While under anesthesia, the area can be moved through a range of motion to distribute the fluid throughout the entire cavity. If arthroscopic equipment is not available, a through-and-through needle lavage can be performed. Isotonic saline can be pressurized and flushed through the synovial structure using a pump or a pressure bag, (Figure 8-13) or by filling the fluid bag with air using a pump or syringe (Figure 8-14). In some cases, it may be best to perform the lavage in a standing horse. The area involved should be anesthetized with local anesthetic prior to flushing.

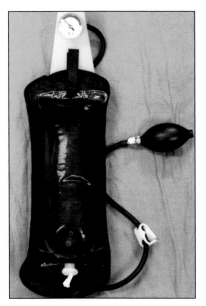

Figure 8-13 One liter pressure bag for performing synovial lavage.

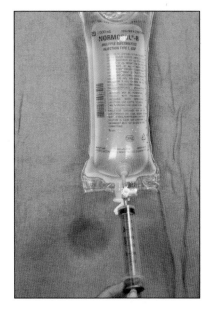

Figure 8-14 Filling fluid bag with air using a syringe for synovial lavage.

🖑 A standing lavage will generally not be as effective as one done under general anesthesia, but is certainly better than not performing a lavage.

🖑 It is important to remember that some joints are very complex and contain multiple joint pouches. All pouches should be lavaged to provide the best chance of success.

🖙 At the end of the lavage, antibiotics can be placed directly into the synovial cavity. The animal should also be started on systemic antibiotics.

🖙 Regional antibiotic perfusion can be performed. See previous topic of heel bulb lacerations for technique.

✓ The wound should be covered with a hypertonic saline dressing that is held in place by antimicrobial roll gauze.

✓ The intra-synovial lavage and regional perfusion can be repeated as needed. As soon as the necrotic debris has been effectively debrided from the wound, a calcium alginate dressing held in place by antimicrobial gauze should be used.

💣 It is generally best not to suture the skin over an open synovial structure until the synovial membrane has healed. Aseptic technique should be used every time the wound is handled to reduce the chance of iatrogenic infection.

Tendon and/or Ligament Lacerations ◉

✔ Lacerations involving tendons or ligaments can be career ending injuries. Appropriate wound care and immobilization are often critical in helping the horse return to athletic function.

✔ Treatment begins with good wound preparation and cleaning followed by an adequate examination of the area.

⌗ The practitioner should be familiar with the anatomy of the flexor and extensor tendons to be able to anticipate what structures are involved (Figure 8-15).

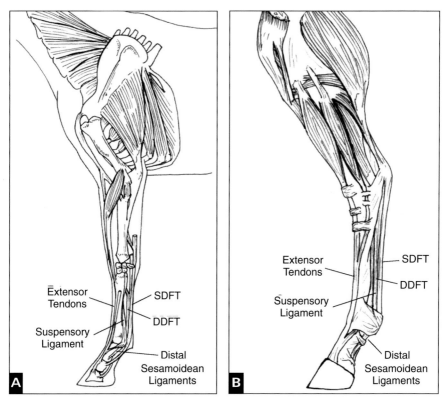

Figure 8-15 Drawing of tendons and ligaments of **A.** front leg, and **B.** hind leg.

💣※ If the laceration is near a tendon sheath, tendon sheath involvement must be ruled out or confirmed. If the tendon sheath is involved, aggressive treatment must be instituted to reduce the occurrence of septic tenosynovitis. See Lacerations of Synovial Structures.

♥ Careful evaluation of the weight bearing leg stance can be helpful in determining if any of the flexor structures are completely transected (Figure 8-16). When the toe comes off the ground, the deep digital flexor may be involved. A dropped fetlock could mean a laceration of the superficial digital flexor tendon or the suspensory ligament. If the animal "knuckles" when it walks, involvement of the extensor tendon should be suspected. The leg should also be picked up and palpated. It is helpful to flex the phalanges to reduce the tension on the flexor tendons. If the superficial digital flexor tendon is intact, the deep digital flexor tendon and suspensory ligament should still be examined.

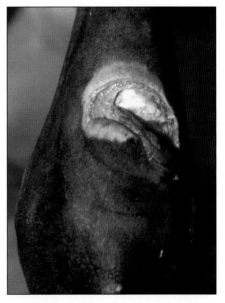

Figure 8-16
Hind leg with partial laceration of the superficial digital flexor tendon.

⚷ If possible, the tendons should be sutured to aid in healing. Multiple techniques have been developed and tested in suturing tendons together. Most of the techniques are quite complex and require significant forethought before beginning the suture line. The two best techniques are the 3-loop pulley and the locking-loop (Figures 8-17 and 8-18). Large diameter non-absorbable suture material is often chosen. With the extended absorption times of synthetic absorbable sutures like Maxon,™ (Tyco Healthcare/Kendall) absorbable sutures can be used as well.

✓ Injuries to the flexor structures are more likely to be career ending than injuries to extensor tendons.

✓ Collateral ligament disruption carries a poor prognosis.

☞ External coaptation of some type will be necessary to support the leg while resting the affected tendon or ligament. If continued wound care is necessary, a splint should be used and appropriate dressings chosen for the stage of wound healing. (See Section 6, Second Intention Healing.) If the wound can be sutured primarily, a cast should be applied. Casts are usually changed every 4 to 6 weeks for a total of 12 to 16 weeks of support. The leg is then kept in a support bandage and splint for 4 to 6 weeks and then another bandage for 4 to 6 weeks.

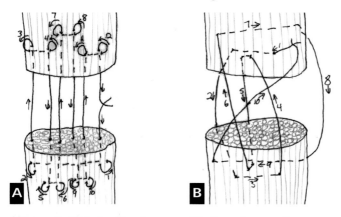

Figure 8-17 A. Locking loop, and **B.** three-loop pulley suture patterns.

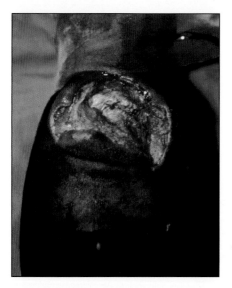

Figure 8-18
The wound in Figure 8-16 after placing locking loop sutures.

Chest Lacerations ⊙

✓ Chest lacerations can penetrate into the pleural cavity leading to a pneumothorax.

🖐 One of the most important steps in treating a chest wound is to confirm or rule out penetration into the pleural space.

☞ Whenever a chest wound is present, the wound must be clipped and aseptically prepared for a thorough examination.

🖐 Aseptic technique should be used when examining all chest wounds until penetration of the pleural cavity can be ruled out. It is helpful to have the room quiet while performing the examination so the practitioner can hear air being sucked into the chest during inspiration.

💣 If the practitioner does not have the facilities or the confidence to place a chest tube, the incision should be closed in as many layers as possible and the horse referred (Figure 8-19).

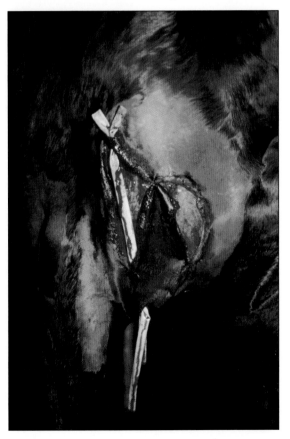

Figure 8-19 Chest wound during closure.

☞ In an emergency situation, a teat cannula can be used to enter the pleural space and a 60 cc syringe with a 3-way stopcock can be used to evacuate the chest. A suction pump will be more efficient and effective.

☞ If possible, a chest tube with a Heimlich valve should be left in place to allow for air evacuation (Figure 8-20). Radiographs can be a useful diagnostic aid in determining if a pneumothorax is present (Figure 8-21). Broad spectrum systemic antibiotics and appropriate wound care should be instituted to reduce the possibility of septic pleuritis. Stent bandages can be sutured over the wound to prevent dehiscence and further pneumothorax.

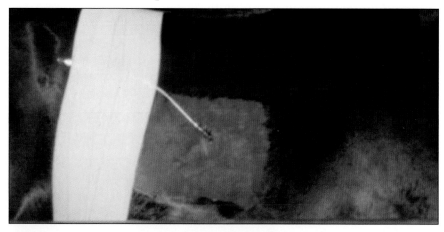

Figure 8-20 Horse with chest wound showing chest tube and Heimlich valve in place.

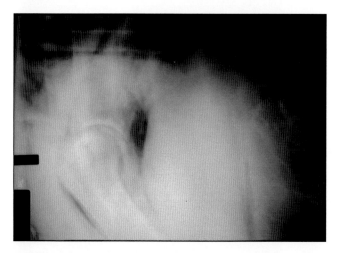

Figure 8-21 Radiograph of horse in Figure 8-20 showing a pneumothorax.

Abdominal Wall Lacerations ⊙

✓ Lacerations to the abdominal wall can be a diagnostic and therapeutic challenge. The abdominal wall is composed of many tissue planes making an accurate diagnosis difficult.

☞ Sterile water-soluble gel should be placed in the wound and the area around the wound clipped. The gel is rinsed out with saline and the obvious necrotic or infected tissue debrided (Figure 8-22). Using aseptic technique, the wound is explored to confirm or rule out penetration into the peritoneal cavity.

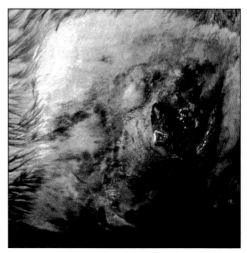

Figure 8-22 Abdominal laceration after clipping.

☞ In some cases where the entry wound is small, the skin should be incised to allow a more complete examination. If necessary, the horse should be sedated. The practitioner must take his or her time and examine all of the tissue planes.

✓ Abdominocentesis can be performed to aid in the diagnosis. An increased protein level or white blood cell count may indicate penetration of the peritoneum. Normal parameters do not rule out penetration.

♥ In many cases, confirmation of peritoneal penetration is not possible and the practitioner must monitor the animal closely in the post-wounding period for signs of peritonitis.

✔ If the wound does not involve the peritoneum, the wound is cleaned and debrided and when possible closed in multiple layers. A drain may be necessary to reduce fluid accumulation (Figure 8-23).

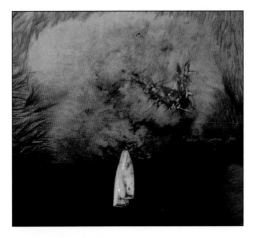

Figure 8-23 Abdominal laceration with penrose drain.

✋ If there has been significant tissue loss in the muscular layers, abdominal herniation is a possible sequela. It is generally not advisable to place a mesh in the immediate post-wounding period. If possible, the wound is treated until healed and a surgical procedure to place a mesh follows.

✔ A "belly-bandage" should be used to support the body wall. While actual support is minimal, the use of a "belly-bandage" will reduce edema formation and will allow for faster healing. There are many types of bandages available including reusable elastic bands (Figure 8-24) and disposable bands made with gauze and elastic bandages (Figure 8-25). In the early stages of the wound when frequent examination is necessary, the reusable elastic bands are best. Broad spectrum antibiotics are useful in the first 3 to 5 days.

⚷ If the wound does involve the peritoneal space a ventral midline celiotomy and abdominal exploration should be performed to adequately treat the animal. A "belly band" should be placed and the animal transported to a facility to allow a complete abdominal exploration.

💣 When peritoneal penetration has occurred, it is possible that there has been trauma to the abdominal viscera. Consequently, the abdomen should be explored and copious lavage performed. Broad spectrum antibiotics should be used to minimize septic peritonitis.

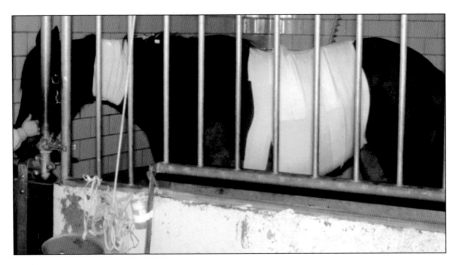

Figure 8-24 Horse with reusable elastic belly-band.

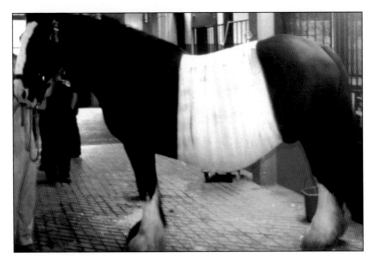

Figure 8-25 Horse with belly band made using roll gauze and elastic bandage material. (Courtesy of Dr. Jennifer MacLeay)

Head Lacerations ⊙

✓ The head is a very complex structure and lacerations can occur anywhere. The good news is that the head has a great vascular supply and wounds generally heal very well. The bad news is that wounds can involve the cranium, eyes, ears, sinuses, salivary ducts, and nares, to name a few structures.

✂ A thorough understanding of the anatomy is critical in helping with an accurate diagnosis.

✓ Radiographs can be used to determine bone involvement in the laceration. However, skull radiographs can be difficult to read with all of the overlapping bones. Wound clipping, cleaning, and digital examination will often guide the practitioner in evaluating bone involvement.

✋ Fractures of the cranium can be challenging but should be considered whenever there is trauma to the caudal aspect of the head. When trauma to the cranium is suspected, a complete neurologic examination should be performed. If the cranium is involved, aggressive therapy should be instituted to stop bacterial penetration and septic encephalitis (Figure 8-26).

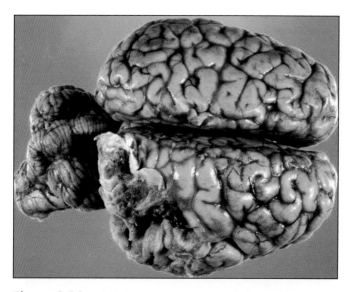

Figure 8-26 Brain after post-mortem evaluation. The horse had hit its head on a feeder penetrating the cranium.

✓ Lacerations around the orbit may involve the structures around the eye as well as the eye itself. A thorough examination of the eye should be performed whenever there is trauma to the surrounding tissues. It is important to use caution when cleaning around the area around the eye to avoid traumatizing the cornea.

💣 Chlorhexidine should not be used around the eye.

✂ Lacerations around the eye should be closed primarily whenever possible to minimize functional problems.

♥ When closing skin lacerations of the eye lids, the practitioner must use small diameter absorbable suture and close the laceration in many layers. Whenever excessive motion is present at the wound closure site, multiple layers of small diameter absorbable suture will minimize the chance of wound dehiscence.

✓ If the cornea has been lacerated, it may require enucleation of the eye.

⚷ Careful evaluation of the surrounding orbit for fractures is another important step in treating lacerations of the eye region. Small bone plates can be used to reconstruct the orbit (Figure 8-27).

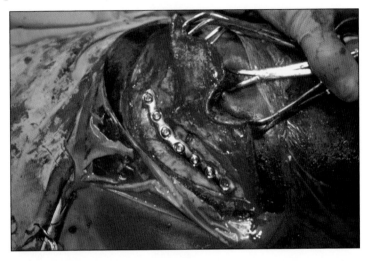

Figure 8-27 Orbit reconstruction using a 3.5 mm reconstruction plate.

✓ Lacerations to the ear provide a particular challenge in cosmetic outcome (Figure 8-28). The ears move through a near 270 degree range of motion and have a cartilage support system.

⚷ Ear lacerations should be treated with primary closure whenever possible.

✋ Ear wounds are rarely too contaminated to close, but they can be too old to hold suture effectively. The collagen in the wound edges is at its weakest point from about 7 days to 20 days after wounding. If the wound fits into this category, it is best to let the wound heal and then reconstruct it at a later date.

⚷ General anesthesia will be required in most cases to achieve the best cosmetic effect. Some type of support can be used in the ear to minimize movement. Rolled-gauze or radiographic film are two examples that have been used in the past.

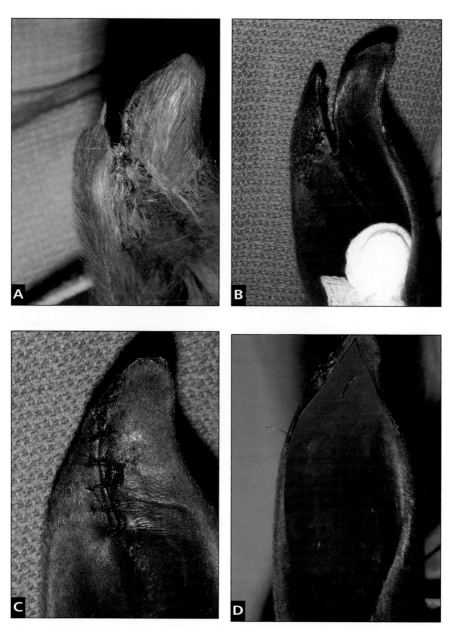

Figure 8-28 A horse with ear laceration. (Courtesy Dr. Gayle Trotter)
A. Presentation. **B.** After clipping and prepping the ear. Note roll gauze in ear to keep prep material from entering ear canal. **C.** After suturing. **D.** With radiographic film sutured to internal aspect of ear to protect against dehiscence.

Trauma to the frontal and maxillary sinuses can lead to fistula formation and bone sequestra so lacerations and trauma to these regions should be treated as soon as possible.

A thorough examination should provide information on bone involvement. If the bone is stable, it can be elevated back into position. If the bone fragments are loose, they should be removed to avoid bone-sequestra formation.

✓ Rotational skin and periosteal flaps may be necessary to treat lacerations where large pieces of bone are removed or missing.

Fistulas can be very difficult to treat.

Lacerations to the mandibular region may involve the salivary ducts. Evaluation of the salivary ducts can be very challenging in horses when significant trauma has occurred. If possible, the integrity of the salivary duct should be determined. If transected, the ends of the salivary duct should be visualized, but this is not always possible. If the cut ends can be visualized, they should be anastomosed. When presented with a chronic laceration of the salivary duct, ablation of the salivary gland should be performed.

✓ Reconstruction of the nares after laceration can be a challenge, but appropriate debridement and effective closure will minimize the chance of incisional dehiscence, encouraging a cosmetic end result.

Lacerations of the nares should be closed in the first 7 days or after 20 days to provide strong collagen in the tissue to hold sutures.

Multiple layers of suture should be used to reduce the chance of incisional dehiscence (Figure 8-29).

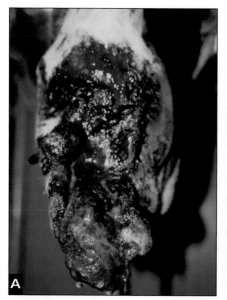

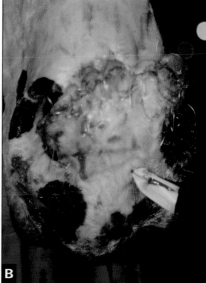

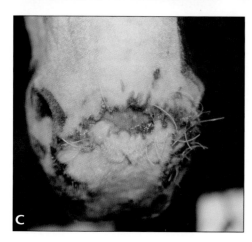

Figure 8-29 A horse with nasal laceration and repair. (Courtesy Dr. Luis Silva) **A.** Presentation. **B.** Closure with size 1 nylon and penrose drain. **C.** 11 days after closure at the time of discharge.

Lacerations of the Axillary Region ⊙

✓ Horses with lacerations of the axillary region will often present with severe sub-cutaneous emphysema (Figure 8-30). The sub-cutaneous emphysema stems from the opening of the wound as the horse advances the leg. As the horse moves forward, the air is pushed up into the sub-cutaneous tissue.

✋ In severe cases, a pneumo-mediastinum can occur and may eventually lead to pneumothorax.

✔ In addition to appropriate wound preparation and exploration, packing the wound and suturing a stent in place will reduce the accumulation of air in the sub-cutaneous space.

✔ Placing the horse in a small stall with an overhead wire will also reduce air accumulation. There is no good way to get rid of the air once it accumulates; it will have to be reabsorbed.

☞ The wound is treated with moist wound-healing principles. Calcium alginate dressings will help to stimulate granulation tissue formation and speed sealing of the wound.

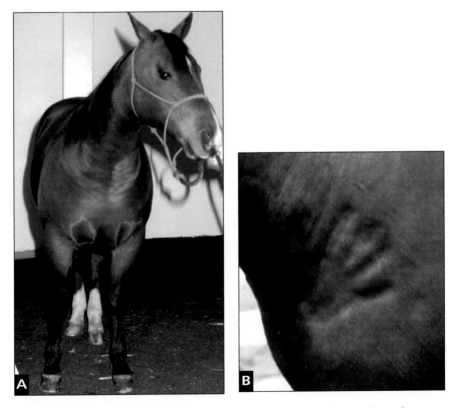

Figure 8-30 A horse with sub-cutaneous emphysema. **A.** Horse from front. **B.** Horse from side showing hand impression still present five minutes later.

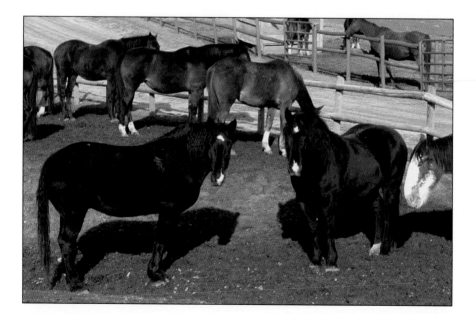

Index

Page numbers followed by an *f* indicate a figure; page numbers followed by a *t* indicate a table.

B

Bacitracin, 39, 40f
  with silver formulations, 38
Back wounds, exploration of, 54
Bacterial colonization, 28
Bacterial infection
  maltrodextran dressing for, 123
  with occlusive dressings, 104-105
  with skin graft, 162
  wound healing and, 32-33
Bacteriology
  for graft infection, 162
  in wound infection, 28-29
Bacteroides fragilis, 123
Ballooning, 92
Basi-sesamoid nerve block, 166
Belly bandage, 184, 185f
Biopsy punches, 152
Biosyn suture material, 76, 77t
Bleach, 37
Blood vessels, severed, 26
Bone
  infection of in non-healin
    wounds, 136-137
  sequestra of, 136
Brain, post-mortem evaluation
  of, 186f
Burn wounds, 101
Butorphanol, 146

C

Calcium alginate, 7
Calcium alginate dressings, 14f,
  105f, 106-107f, 116-117
  for axillary lacerations, 191
  with dry wound, 118-120
  with moist wound, 121-122
  in moist wound healing, 110
  in pad and rope, 118f
Cannon region/bone
  anatomy of, 60t, 61f

surgical tubing on, 95f
ultrasound at level of, 66f
Cannon wound
  calcium alginate dressing on, 119f
  distal, 27f
  semi-occlusive foam dressings
    for, 127-130
Carpal canal
  contrast radiograph of, 67f
  ultrasound of foreign material
    in, 66f
Carpal wound, 27f, 50f
  primary closure of, 70-71f
Carpus
  after carpal arthroscopy, 112f
  anatomy of, 62t, 63f
  palpating wound at, 65f
Cast
  after grafting, 159, 161f
  after primary wound closure, 71f
  after skin graft, 163
  application of in primary wound
    closure, 88
  complications of, 159
  for heel bulb laceration, 168-170
  for hoof wall avulsion, 173
  slipper, 168-169f
  for tendon and ligament
    lacerations, 180
Cast material splints, 19
Caustic agents, 134
Celiotomy, midline, 184
Cellophane, sterilized, 101
Cephalosporin, 170
Chemical debridement, 37
Chemical trauma, 30
Chemotactic agents, 126-127
Chemotactic factors
  in moist wound healing, 101
  release of, 46
Chest drain, 56, 73f

physical, 6, 43

sharp, 7, 42

for excess granulation tissue, 134

Dermatome harvesting, 155-156

Detomidine

hypotension with, 26

for skin grafting sedation, 146

Devitalized tissue, 46

Dexamethasone, 131

Digital palpation, synovial structure, 175

Digital tendon sheath, 176f

injection of, 59f

Disposable diapers, 9, 10f

Distal leg splint, 20f

Donor sites, skin graft, 145

closure of, 150f

punch grafts within, 151f

Dorsal spinous process wound, 8f

Drains

for abdominal wall lacerations, 184f

ascending infection with, 72

in chest wound, 56, 73f

for nasal laceration, 190f

passive and active, 72

positioning of, 72

Dressing manufacturers, 132t

Dressings, 23

for absorption, 9-10

for axillary lacerations, 191

for cleaning and prepping, 4-5

for compression, 11

for debridement, 6-7

flow chart for selecting, 133f

gauze, 103

for heel bulb laceration, 170, 171f

methods of applying, 14-15

for moisture, 14

non-adherent, 103, 104

for packing, 7-8

with primary wound closure, 87

for protection, 13

recommendations for, 133f

in second-intention healing, 100, 103-132

semi-occlusive foam, 105f

silver impregnated, 38

for skin grafts

frequency of changes in, 159

primary and secondary, 160f

selection of, 158

in wound immobilization, 159

for support, 12

topical, 122-123, 124f

transparent nylon, 101

wet-to-dry and dry-to-dry, 43

Dry wound dressings, 118-120

E

Ear

clipping and prepping of, 188f

lacerations of, 188f

wounds of, 187

Edema, abdominal wall, 184

Elastic adhesive dressing, 149

Elastic bandage

for abdominal wall lacerations, 184, 185f

for heel bulb laceration, 168

in skin graft, 160f

Elastic wraps, application of, 15

Emergency transport, 19-21

Emphysema, sub-cutaneous, 190, 191f

Endoscopy, 54

Enzymatic debridement, 46-47

Epidermal growth factor, 126

Epithelialization, 126

in punch grafting, 153

slowing process of, 134

Eschmarch's bandage, 95f

NOTES

NOTES

Recommended Readings

Ashcroft GS, Mills SJ. *Androgen receptor-mediated inhibition of cutaneous wound healing.* J. Clin Invest 110:615-624, 2002.

Berry DB, Sullins KE. *Effects of topical application of antimicrobials and bandaging on healing and granulation tissue formation in wounds of the distal aspect of the limbs in horses.* Am J Vet Res 64:88-92, 2003.

Bigbie RB, Schumacher J, Swaim SF, Purohit RC, Wright JC. *Effects of amnion and live yeast cell derivative on second-intention healing in horses.* Am J. Vet Res 52:1376-1382, 1991.

Bloom H. *Cellophane dressing for second degree burns.* Lancet 2:559, 1945.

Booth JH, Benrimoj SI, Nimmo GR. *In vitro interactions of neomycin sulfate, bacitracin, and polymyxin B sulfate.* Int J Dermatol 33:517-520, 1994.

Boyce ST, Warden GD, Holder IA. *Cytotoxicity testing of topical antimicrobial agents on human deratinocytes and fibroblasts for cultured skin grafts.* J Burn Care Rehabil 16:97-103, 1995.

Bull JP, Squire JR, Topley E. *Experiments with occlusive dressings of a new plastic.* Lancet 2:213-214, 1948.

Carter CA, Jolly DG, Worden CE, Hendren DG, Kane CJM. *Platelet-rich plas~ ,el promotes differentiation and regeneration during equine wound healing perit., al and Molecular Pathology.* In Press 2003.

Cohen MA, Eaglstein WH. *Recomb.n gut human platelet-derived growth factor gel speeds healing of act.te , "-th; \,;e-s punch biopsy wounds.* J Am Acad Dermatol 45:857-862, 2001.

Geronemus RG, Mertz PM, Eaglestein WH. *Wound healing: The effects of topical antimicrobial agents.* Arch Dermatol 115:1311-1314, 1979.

Goodrich LR, Moll HD, Crisman MV. Lessard P, Bigbie RB. *Comparison of equine amnion and a nonadherent wound dressing material for bandaging pinch-grafted wounds in ponies.* Am J Vet Res 61:326-329, 2000.

Hansbrough JF, Achauer B, Dawson J, Himel H, Luterman A, Slater H, Levenson S, Salzberg CA, Hansbrough WB, Dore C. *Wound healing in partial thickness burn wounds treated with collangenase ointment versus silver sulfadiazine cream.* J Burn Care Rehabil 16:241-247, 1995.

Hashimoto I, Nakanishi H, Shono Y, Toda M, Hidetaka T, Arase S. *Angiostatic effects of corticosteroid on wound healing of the rabbit ear.* J Med Invest 49:61-66, 2002.

Hohn DC, Granelli SG, Burton RW, Hunt TK. *Antimicrobial systems of the surgical wound — 11 detection of antimicrobial protein in cell free wound fluid.* Am J Surg 113:601-606, 1977.

Katz MH, Alvarez AF, Dirsner RS, Eaglstein WH, Falanga V. *Human wound fluid from acute wounds stimulates fibroblast and endothelial cell growth.* J Am Acad Dermatol 25:1054-1058, 1991.

We hope you enjoy this
Made Easy Series volume for the
Equine Practitioner.
If you would like more information on
other **Made Easy** Series
products please call 877-306-9793
or visit our online store at
www.veterinarywire.com

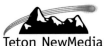

Teton NewMedia
P.O. Box 4833, Jackson, WY 83001

WOUND CARE MANAGEMENT
for the Equine Practitioner

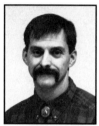

A Must Have for the Equine Port–A–Vet Library

- A liberally illustrated guide to traditional and advanced wound healing techniques (247 figures, 40 in color).

- Detailed guidelines for basic wound cleaning, preparation and closure including bandaging and grafting techniques.

- Practical coverage of moist wound healing concepts and techniques.

Dean A. Hendrickson DVM, MS

- Important anatomical considerations are emphasized by body region.

CD-ROM Features:

- 25 case studies, 4 QuickTime™ videos, 3 QuickTime™ Virtual Reality images, and many additional still images featuring different bandaging, casting and moist wound healing techniques and outcomes.

- Windows® and MacOS Compatible, html files run using your internet browser program. The CD-ROM is best viewed with your screen resolution set at 1024 by 768 pixels or better. QuickTime™ 5 or newer is needed to play the videos on this CD-ROM.

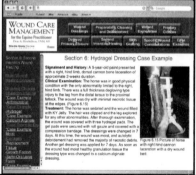

Published titles in the **Made Easy** Series
for the Equine Practitioner
Ophthalmology • Broodmare Reproduction

Forthcoming titles in the **Made Easy** Series
for the Equine Practitioner
Dermatology

Innovative
Publishing

QuickTime™

Windows is a registered trademark of Microsoft Corporation.
MacOS and Quicktime are registered trademarks of Apple Computer, Inc.

ISBN 159161022-2

9 781591 610229

1-591610-22-2 (CD+Book)